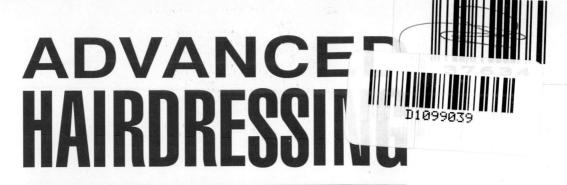

ADVANCED HAIRDRESSING

SECOND EDITION

A coursebook for Level 3

STEPHANIE HENDERSON
Cert Ed, LCGI

and JANETTE CHIVELL
Cert Ed

First published in 1997 by:
Stanley Thornes (Publishers) Ltd
Second edition 1999

Reprinted in 2002 by:
Nelson Thornes Ltd
Delta Place
27 Bath Road
CHELTENHAM
GL53 7TH
United Kingdom

02 03 04 05 06 / 10 9 8 7 6 5 4 3

A catalogue record for this book is available from the British Library

ISBN 0 7487 5165 3

Cover photograph by Laurence Bulaitis
Hair by Uxbridge College Artistic Team, Kirsten Harjette and Stephanie Linton
Make-up by Claudia Gardner

Page make-up by Columns Design Ltd

Printed in Great Britain by Scotprint

Contents

This chapter includes all the required knowledge for Unit 15, which
applies to loading the work of teams and individuals to achieve objectives

Acknowledgements

The authors and publishers wish to thank the following for permission to reproduce material:

BLM Health – photograph of pediculosis capitis (eggs) on page 18

Goldwell – photographs of smooth cuticles, damaged cuticles and fragilitis crinium on page 16

St John's Institute of Dermatology, London – photographs of tinea capitis (ringworm) and scabies on page 17; impetigo on page 18

Institute of Trichology and the International Association of Trichologists – photographs of alopecia areata, trichorrhexis nodosa and psoriasis on page 16; pediculosis capitis (head louse) and folliculitis on page 18

Redken Laboratories Ltd – photograph of monilethrix on page 16

Nyxon – photograph of Afro tongs, page 136

Wella Great Britain – pages 6, 75, 111 and 152. Credits for page 6:

- Hair by Brendan O'Sullivan for Regis at Wella
- Photography by Trevor Leighton
- Make-up by Cheryl Phelps-Gardiner

Uxbridge College Training Salons – photographs on pages 51 (middle), 59, 134, 151, 154, 155, 173, 185, 186, colour plates 1–8

- Uxbridge College Artistic Team, Jan Chivell (Perms, Colours & Styling), Antonella Desiano (Cuts), Stephanie Henderson (Styling), Jo Kearvell (Cuts), Laine Russell and Sarah Steadman (Styling), Karen Overy (Cut, Styling & Make-up), Amisha Vadher (Cut & Styling)

Sam Richardson (photography) and Zöe Irwin (hair), pages 47, 51 (top), 62, 78, 125, 126, 129, 139, 147, 148

Gary Lee – photographs on page 49

Samantha Fox of Martin Gold, Stanmore – photograph (left) on page 126

Neville Daniel; hair by Errol Douglas – photograph on page 129

Laurence Bulaitis – photographs on page 137

Errol Douglas – photograph on page 133

Salon Publicity (Giannini Studios) – photograph on page 156

All original cartoons by Derek Gibbons

Thanks to David Brown for technical assistance and to Annette Cost for appraisal training

Introduction

This book is designed as a guide for hairdressers undertaking the City & Guilds/Hairdressing Training Board National, or Scottish, Vocational Qualification at Level 3. It is also intended for those wishing to enhance their technical hairdressing skills and expand their knowledge of the non-technical aspects of hairdressing, such as the roles and responsibilities of salon staff.

Advanced Hairdressing follows on from *Basic Hairdressing* by Stephanie Henderson. Written in an easy-to-follow style, it covers not only fashion styling, creative perming and colouring techniques but also health and safety within the salon, client care and consultation, training and assessing methods and techniques, along with ways of making your salon financially successful and promoting its staff and services.

The role of a salon supervisor or manager can often include training and assessing staff who are working towards City & Guilds Vocational Qualifications at Levels 1 and 2. This assessment takes place against national standards set by the industry training organisation. Within the NVQ Level 3 framework, City & Guilds offers the opportunity to gain TDLB D32 and D33 awards, which are designed to enable assessors within the hairdressing industry to assess candidates' performances fairly and reliably. Chapters 12 and 13 cover these areas in full, giving a step-by-step guide to the requirements candidates must meet in order to qualify for the awards.

Chapter 14 discusses how to enable both individuals and hairdressing teams to become better at their jobs through careful management strategies. Chapter 10 shows how to lead teams to achieve their goals such as putting on promotions and shows.

Hairdressing is a creative industry which allows individuals to progress through a variety of levels or stages. Within the industry, a wide range of opportunities exist, from stylist to salon manager or owner, from freelance or session work to work in the theatre or television, and from technical work for product manufacturers to involvement in education and training. Whichever area you see as your goal, a thorough understanding of all aspects of the hairdressing profession is essential, and this book will be a valuable guide.

1 Client care

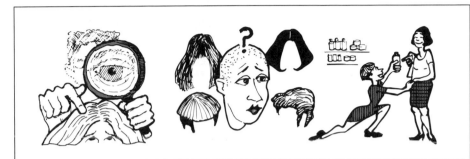

Client consultation

Remember
Clients may have no idea of what salon service they want. The consultation is your opportunity to make your recommendations and to build up a good relationship, which may lead to a return visit.

Client consultation means talking to your client and giving advice before starting work on their hair.

During this consultation you will also be examining your client's hair by brushing it through. In the same way that doctors diagnose their patients' illnesses, you will be able to diagnose any hair or scalp conditions and take the appropriate action.

You will also be able to assess the client's requirements generally, and make recommendations for a hairstyle to suit their appearance and lifestyle.

HEALTH MATTERS
Standing all day long
Shoulders   Work with your shoulders relaxed. Exercise helps by contracting and relaxing the muscles. Try raising your shoulders up towards your ears and letting them drop. Do this six times in ten seconds, and repeat at least twice a day.

Gaining information

You must find out:

- The client's name
- The service (e.g. cut, perm, colour) required
- The chosen hairstyle (you may need to use a style book)

Don't forget that all salon **records** are **confidential** (those kept on a computer are covered by the **Data Protection Act** 1984) and must not be accessed without your supervisor's permission. This includes client records and staff records such as CVs, staff appraisals and disciplinary procedures.

1

Record keeping

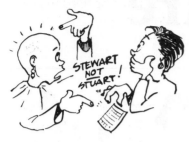

Why bother to keep client records?

- A new stylist will be able to attend to a client **when the normal stylist is away** (off sick or on holiday).
- It is possible to check **when the client last visited your salon** for a colour or a perm (some salons send out reminder cards).
- Clients feel they are being **professionally treated** when they see you are checking their personal records.
- You are able to know exactly what **perm lotion** was used at which strength and what curler size was used on previous occasions (especially useful if the perm was too tight or too soft). Records of **relaxers** – the product, strength and development time – must also be recorded as they are particularly strong chemicals.
- You are able to know what make of **colour** or **bleach** was used on previous occasions, which colour was used, the peroxide strength and how long the hair took to process.
- Records of **conditioning treatments** will allow you to know how many were needed before the hair returned to good condition.
- You can keep details of any **special conditions**, such as any medication the client has been taking, or details of a resistant section of hair.
- You can deal with **complaints** more efficiently. For example, if a client complains that a perm has not lasted, but your records show that the perm used was a very soft one which was only intended to last six to eight weeks, you can remind the client of the details.
- You will have a record of the client's **telephone number** and **address**, which may be needed if an appointment has to be changed.

Records are generally kept for perming, hair colouring and bleaching, and for conditioning treatments.

Remember

If client records are held on computer your company must be registered with the Data Protection Register. The information must be accurate and not open to misuse. Clients must have access to information if they request it.

Example of a record card

Client name					Special notes		
Address					Homecare sales		
Daytime tel. no.							
Date	Stylist	Scalp condition	Hair condition	Technique	Products	Development time	Results

Record cards

These are stored either in a filing box or in a filing cabinet, in alphabetical order according to the surname of the client. Cards must be filled in and replaced in alphabetical order after use. Some salons design their own record cards; others buy or use specially made cards.

Computers

Many salons now use computers, not only for recording takings but also for keeping client records. To use a computer properly, you need training. All computers are operated by a program, which is known as the **software**. Salon computer software will be used to classify, store and retrieve information: the type of software used to do this is known as a **database**.

Once all client records are on the database, retrieving the information is quick and easy.

Client consultation

Remember

All consultations are done on dry hair before shampooing. You cannot always see the problems (e.g. dry ends) when the hair is wet.

Experienced hairdressers will be able to produce a perfect hairstyle for each individual client by considering:

- Face shape (oval, round, long or square)
- Approximate height (tall or short)
- Approximate size (thin or overweight)
- Approximate age (not everyone can take young styles)
- Skin colour
- Lifestyle (busy people want a hairstyle that is quick and easy to manage)
- Personality (quiet and shy or lively and outgoing)
- Occupation (some professions may have strict rules about hair length)
- Cost (make sure a price list is accessible)
- Medical history (some illnesses affect perming and tinting)
- Occasion (dinner dance, wedding)
- Time available (can the client spare the time for a long process such as perming?)

All this should be done **before** gowning up the client so that you can consider their clothes and lifestyle, and see their height and body shape more clearly.

Allow enough **time** to complete your consultation checklist.

Client communications

Verbal communication

Most hairdressers are **excellent communicators**, because they develop good verbal skills through continued client contact. They build up relationships with clients based on quality of service and professional advice, by always promoting accurate information.

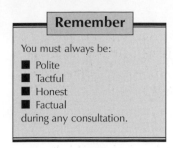

During the **initial consultation** you must ensure that you **accurately establish your client's wishes**, and that the client **understands and agrees to** what is **finally decided**. If you feel that the client is still unclear, then repeat a summary of the main information. Your communication skills are just as important when working with new clients as with regular clients, always promoting a **professional salon image**.

Listen to your client. Many clients never return to a salon because, although they may have been given a lovely new hairstyle, it was not the one they asked for!

Sample questions for clients
Here are some examples of questions to ask your clients:

- *'How often do you shampoo your hair?'*
  If the answer is 'every day', the client probably has greasy hair and scalp.

- *'How have you been lately?'*
  This gives the client a chance to tell you if they are taking any medication that may affect their hair condition.

- *'Do you have your hair permed or coloured?'*
  The client can then tell you about any chemicals they may have used on their hair.

Benefits of carrying out a good consultation
- Repeat business: **a satisfied client will tell a few people about you, but an unhappy client will tell everyone**.
- It will promote your salon's **professional image**.
- It will **encourage clients to take up** both **existing services** (such as perming and colouring) and **new services** that they may not have tried before, such as conditioning treatments combined with head and shoulder massages.

Consequences of not carrying out consultations correctly
The client may not only be dissatisfied with the service (for example, if her new style was difficult to keep because you had not suggested a light perm), but you could **potentially damage** the hair or scalp by failing to notice adverse hair or scalp conditions such as cuts or abrasions on the scalp before applying perm lotion.

Salon business and potential promotion could be lost because of misinterpretation of the client's wishes. This could lead to mistrust, arguments and embarrassment.

Developing and responding to non-verbal clues

There are other ways of responding to your client as well as talking to them. People communicate **non-verbally** all the time, using both appearance and gestures.

Appearance
Hairdressing is all about creating images. Remember, not everyone wants a new hairstyle whenever they visit the salon. Many clients are quite happy for you to maintain the style they have, possibly with a few variations.

Personal hygiene

You will either be sitting or standing **very close to your client** during your consultation as well as when doing their hair, so remember that both **bad breath** (especially if you smoke and your client does not) and **body odour** can offend. Keep your breath fresh and remember that soap and water will remove stale sweat, whilst deodorants (which mask smells) and anti-perspirants (which reduce sweating) can help to prevent body odour.

Remember to keep your **hands and fingernails** clean and well presented. Nothing looks worse than chipped nail polish in the mirror as you are doing their hair! You are selling personal image and style to your clients. That means you have to lead the way.

Gestures

The obvious gestures that you should look for when selling products and services are:

Head nodding

This means that a client is listening to what you are saying with agreement. A slow single nod means you should continue what you are saying; several quick nods means that the client wants to interrupt or make a comment of their own.

Eye contact

By looking into someone's eyes you can soon see if they are feeling friendly or hostile towards you. When you are selling to clients, look them in the eye while speaking to them to gain their confidence.

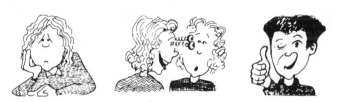

Smiling

Simply occasionally smiling at clients will automatically create good humour in the salon. It is very difficult not to smile back at someone who smiles at you!

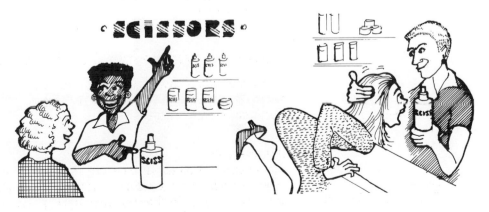

Developments in technology

Hairdressing is a fashion industry that is constantly changing. In order to be able to create the latest styles you must be able to use the most up-to-date tools and equipment and the most recently launched products.

To maintain your awareness of both current and emerging fashion trends and the latest developments in technology you should:

- Read **trade publications** such as *The Hairdressers' Journal*, *Your Salon* or *Esoterica*.
- Read **general hair and beauty magazines** such as *Vogue* or *Hair* which are available to the general public.
- Attend **seminars** and **training courses**, either **'in-house'** at the salon or **externally at** a local college/private training centre/manufacturers' training school or hairdressing wholesalers.
- Attend **trade events** such as the hair shows at Wembley, London.
- Attend **hair and fashion shows** such as the World Congress in London, the Alternative Hair Show and others in the UK and around the world
- Watch **television**, not only for informative current programmes, but by using your video to watch some of the many **training videos** available.

Once you have this knowledge you should be able to:

- **Offer the most up-to-date advice and the most complete range of services to clients.**
- **Know where to access new products/equipment needed in the future.**
- **Access new training courses to be able to keep up with the latest developments.**

Remember

Be prepared!
It is better to be practised and competent with new products and materials beforehand rather than have to turn clients away.

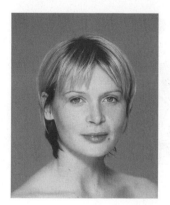 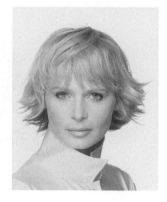

Before and after: 'Headlines' – a recent styling innovation from Wella

To do

- Describe how you could keep pace with recent developments in:
  - Cutting
  - Colouring
  - Perming
  - Conditioning treatments and massage
  - African/Afro-Caribbean
  - Long hair dressing
  - Photographic work
  - Motivating your staff
  - Health and Safety
  - Interviewing techniques
  - Show work and promotions

Examining the hair and scalp

Finding out what the client wants to have done to their hair and choosing a style is very important, but sometimes the client's hair and scalp condition limits the range of services you are able to offer them.

For instance, if the hair is untreated it means that no chemicals have been used on it, but if it has been chemically treated it will react differently to blow-drying and setting, perming, colouring and bleaching.

To undertake a hair and scalp analysis you need to section the hair in a 'hot cross bun' format, from ear to ear and from nape to front hairline. Then take each section about one inch deep horizontally across the two quarter sections at the back, repeating the inspection to the front (in the same way as stylists generally section off to apply tint to regrowth areas). This will allow you to observe both the **scalp** and the **full length of the hair** on different areas of the head.

A temporary colour (a coloured mousse or setting lotion) affects different parts of the hair from a permanent colour (a tint). You will need to recognise the different parts of the hair and learn how they are affected by various chemicals, and whether coloured hair can be permed, coloured or bleached in future.

HEALTH MATTERS

Standing all day long

Legs   Many hairdressers suffer from varicose veins, especially if they have had children. This is because you are not moving your legs when you are standing still and the blood does not circulate properly back to the heart. The result can be both swollen ankles and varicose veins (because the veins have become full of blue, de-oxygenated blood).

If it is impossible to take a rest at work with your feet up, make sure that you do it at home by raising your feet on a stool or chair.

Exercise is the best way to prevent varicose veins. If you cannot walk or cycle to work, then try exercising in the evenings or on your day off. Walking is an excellent form of exercise.

Hair can be damaged by chemical treatments. It can also be damaged by handling – bad brushing, excessive blow-drying or tonging. Again, you will need to know what part of the hair is damaged and whether further services can be carried out.

As you are carrying out your consultation you can start to diagnose your client's hair condition. In order to understand why some people have shiny, manageable hair in good condition while others have very difficult hair, you need to know more about hair structure.

Hair structure

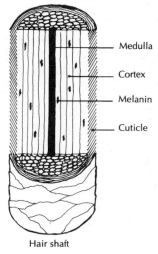

Longitudinal section of a hair

Each hair is made up of three layers – rather like a pencil.

- The outside layer, the **cuticle**, is thin and flat (like the paint on a pencil).
- The middle layer, the **cortex**, is the strong, main part of the hair (like the wood of the pencil).
- The central layer, the **medulla**, runs finely through the middle (like the lead in a pencil).

The cuticle

If you look carefully at the diagrams you will see that the cuticle is actually made up of **overlapping scales** (7–10 layers). These scales look like the tiles on a roof, with the edges all lying away from the scalp. They are translucent, like frosted glass, so that the hair colour (in the cortex) can be seen through them.

This outside layer of the hair shaft is very tough and holds the whole hair together, but it may be damaged by strong chemicals (such as perms or bleaches) or harsh treatments (such as over back-brushing).

If the cuticle scales have been damaged or broken and have opened up, and chemicals have been absorbed into the cortex, the hair surface will look and feel rough and dull like sandpaper. If the scales are undamaged and closed tight and flat then the hair will appear beautifully shiny like glass.

The cortex

The cortex is the main part of the hair, lying underneath the cuticle. Hairdressers need to understand the cortex because this is where all the changes take place when hair is blow-dried, set, permed, tinted or bleached.

It is made from many strands or fibres (the alpha-helix shape), which are twisted together like knitting wool. These can stretch, then return to their original length.

Hair is made of a protein called **keratin**, itself made up from amino acid units, which are found in long coiled chains called **polypeptide chains**. All the coils of polypeptide chains are held together by various links and bonds.

Look at the diagram on page 9 and find the **temporary bonds**. These are the **hydrogen bonds** and **salt links**. They break and rejoin whenever hair is blow dried, set, tonged or hot brushed into a different style. They are called temporary bonds because all these processes can be easily reversed by dampening the hair and starting again.

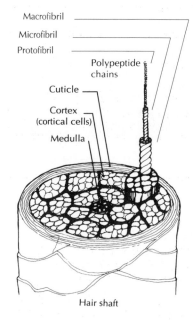

Cross-section of a hair

There are also permanent bonds in the diagram: these are called **disulphide bonds**. Disulphide bonds are very strong and can be broken only by using a strong chemical on the hair such as permanent wave lotion.

The cortex also contains all the **colour pigments** in the hair. These pigments are called **melanin** (brown/black) and **pheomelanin** (yellow/red).

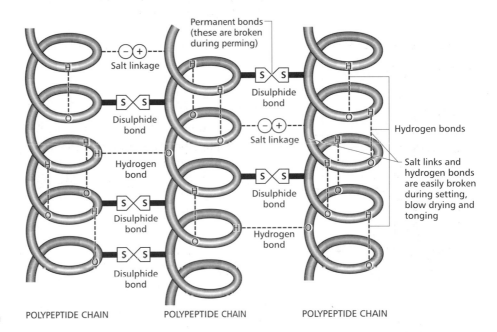

The structure of keratin

The medulla

The medulla does not have any real function. It is not always present in scalp hairs, particularly if the hair is fine.

To do

■ Sketch the diagram of the hair structure and label it (without looking at this book).
■ Make a list of all the technical words related to hair structure that you have just learned and explain them in your own way.
■ Copy the diagram of the structure of keratin, then try to draw in and name the links and bonds (without looking at this book).

Scalp (or skin) structure

There are two main types of hair on the human body. Fine **vellus hair** grows on the body; stronger **terminal hair** grows on the scalp and makes up eyebrows, eyelashes, beards and moustaches. A third type of hair, **lanugo hair**, is only found on human fetuses and is even finer than vellus hair. The scalp is stronger than the rest of the body skin (which is why we can put chemicals on scalp hair without causing too much damage) but its structure is otherwise similar to body skin.

The structure of the skin

Hair is made of the protein keratin, which is dead. There are no nerve endings inside hair and so it does not hurt when we cut through it, or when chemicals such as perm lotions or bleaches are put onto it.

However, we can feel someone pulling our hair because it is attached to the scalp by its root, sitting in a tiny pocket called the **hair follicle**. Nerve endings attached to the hair root tell us when our hair is being pulled and when a hair should stand on end. We all have occasional 'goose pimples', when our hair stands on end if we are very cold or frightened. The **arrector pili** muscle is attached to the hair root and contracts (or squeezes together) to pull the hair upright, creating the goose pimples.

The **sebaceous gland** is also attached to the hair follicle and produces **sebum**, the hair's natural oil or lubricant. The sebum flows around the hair root and outwards onto the scalp surface. If too much sebum is produced, the scalp and hair will be too greasy, but if too little sebum is produced the hair and scalp will be too dry.

The scalp (and skin) is divided into two layers:

● The outer layer – the **epidermis** – is the outer protective layer of skin. It is constantly shedding itself, losing dead skin cells. When this happens excessively on the scalp it is known as **dandruff**.

● The inner layer – the **dermis** – is the thickest and most important part of the skin. It is where the hair follicles, nerve endings, sebaceous glands, blood supply and sweat glands are found.

Hair could not grow without its own blood supply. The heart pumps blood containing food and oxygen (needed to make new keratin) through our arteries towards the skin surface. The arteries become **small blood capillaries** in the dermis, where they supply blood into the bottom of the hair root or follicle to feed the **dermal papilla**. The more blood flowing towards the hair papilla, the more the hair will grow. Therefore, when our skin is red and warm in the summer our hair (and nails) grow quicker.

We can also regulate our body temperature through our skin because we have **sweat glands**. These produce **sweat**, which flows on to our skin through our pores, cooling us down as it evaporates.

To do

■ Copy the diagram of the scalp and skin structure and then try to label it on your own without looking at this book.
■ Describe the structure of the scalp or skin in your own words.

Ethnic structural hair types

There are three main racial differences in hair type:

● European (**Caucasian**) hair is generally wavy.
● Asian (**Mongoloid**) hair is usually straight.
● Negroid (**African/Afro-Caribbean**) hair is usually curly.

European and Asian hair (typically very straight hair found in people of Chinese and Japanese origin) react in much the same way to chemical treatments, but you will need to read Chapter 8, 'African/Afro-Caribbean hair', for details of this hair structure and how it responds to relaxing treatments.

Hair growth and life cycle

Hair grows from the bottom of its root at the dermal papilla, where new cells are constantly being produced. These soft cells become hardened to form strong hair above the skin surface. The average rate of hair growth is 1.25 cm ($\frac{1}{2}$ in.) per month. This is what keeps hairdressers in business!

There are approximately 100,000 hairs growing on the average scalp, and there is a constant daily loss of 50–100 scalp hairs. We lose these hairs because every so often the hair follicle has a period of rest, and so the hair falls out.

The growing stage of the hair is called the **anagen** stage. When the hair starts to go into its resting state, it is said to be in the **catagen** stage. The resting stage is called the **telogen** stage.

Obviously not all hairs rest at the same time – or we would all be bald!

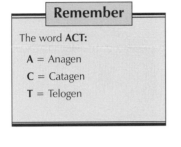

Remember

The word **ACT:**

A = Anagen

C = Catagen

T = Telogen

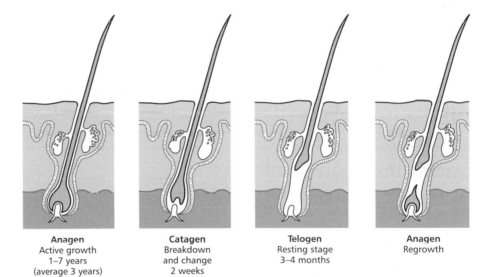

Anagen	Catagen	Telogen	Anagen
Active growth 1–7 years (average 3 years)	Breakdown and change 2 weeks	Resting stage 3–4 months	Regrowth

The hair growth cycle

The diagram above shows how the hair gradually stops growing and starts again.

Each hair grows for between $1\frac{1}{4}$ and 7 years before reaching a resting stage. This means that some clients' hair will grow to shoulder length:

$$1\frac{1}{4} \text{ years} \times 1.25 \text{ cm } (\tfrac{1}{2} \text{ in.}) \text{ per month} = 18.75 \text{ cm } (7\tfrac{1}{2} \text{ in.})$$

but other clients' hair will grow down to their waist or longer:

$$7 \text{ years} \times 1.25 \text{ cm } (\tfrac{1}{2} \text{ in.}) \text{ per month} = 105 \text{ cm } (42 \text{ in.})$$

So when a client complains that they cannot grow long hair you can explain to them that it is because their hair has a short life cycle.

Hair thickness

Remember

Some people have very fine hair, but plenty of it, while some people have very coarse hair but not very much of it.

This is known as hair texture, and it is determined by the thickness of each individual hair, i.e. whether it is coarse, medium or fine.

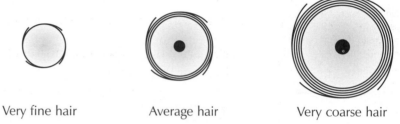

Very fine hair   Average hair   Very coarse hair

To do

- Pull out three hairs from your head: one from the front, the middle and the back.
- Ask several friends to do the same.
- Compare the thickness of each individual hair against a sheet of paper.

Establishing hair condition

Hair in good condition will shine and look great. Clients with a new haircut and this type of hair will also find that perms, colours and highlights take equally well.

Internal and external hair condition

Location	Good condition	Poor condition
Surface condition	Cuticle scales lie flat and close together.	Cuticle scales are raised and open, sometimes damaged. Surface is rough and dull, e.g. fragilitis crinium (split ends). Damaged cuticle. This is known as **porous hair**.
Internal condition	Surface is smooth and shiny. The chemical links and bonds in keratin within the cortex are strong and elastic and contain natural moisture.	The chemical links and bonds in keratin within the cortex have been broken by strong chemicals, e.g. perm lotion, hydrogen peroxide. This hair has lost strength, elasticity and moisture (through the open cuticle scales). This is known as **over-elastic** hair (stretchy hair).

However, hair that is damaged and dry may need special perm lotions or different types of colorants to improve its condition.

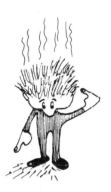

Remember

- **Physical handling** damage is caused by bad brushing and combing (over back-combing) or excessive drying (hairdriers too hot, excessive tonging or hot brushing).
- **Weather damage** is caused by excessive exposure to the sun, sea and wind.
- **Chemical damage** is caused by excessive perming, bleaching (highlighting) and tinting.

Remember

Always be tactful when dealing with incorrectly treated hair. Everyone makes the odd mistake, so be positive and helpful towards your client.

Physical and handling damage

Here are some causes of physical and handling damage:

- **Bad brushing** – disentangling from the roots instead of the ends.
- **Bad combing** – over back-combing.
- **Over-drying** – the hairdrier too hot and held too close to the hair.
- Excessive use of **electrical appliances** – tongs and hot brushes.
- **Excessive tension** – especially from rubber bands.
- **Strong sunlight, sea and chlorinated water** – hair lightens/dries out.
- **Very windy conditions** – cause hair to tangle.

Chemical damage

You already know what chemically damaged hair looks like, but you need to know why the damage may have happened. For instance, a perm could look straight either because it was overprocessed (a straight frizz) or because it was underprocessed. The underprocessed perm could possibly be re-permed but the hair of an overprocessed perm would be sure to disintegrate and break off if further perming was attempted.

The general reasons why hair may be chemically damaged are:

- Clients have used products from the chemist **without any professional skill** or knowledge.
- The hairdresser has not carried out a **proper consultation** or analysis.
- The hairdresser has **misinterpreted** the client's requirements.
- The hairdresser did not have enough **practical skill, product or technical knowledge**.
- The product was **applied badly**, left on too long (overprocessed), or not long enough (underprocessed).

Some specific reasons for chemical damage are:

- **Perming** – hair looks frizzy and may break off (the scalp may be sore or burned).
- **Relaxing** – curly hair has been permanently straightened and is starting to break off.
- **Bleaching and highlighting** – hair looks and feels 'straw-like' and the colour may be patchy.

- **Tinting** (tint applied on top of tint) – the hair feels very dry and the colour is patchy and uneven.
- **Colour strippers** – hair may be patchy in colour if strippers are not applied quickly and evenly.

Test your knowledge

State the effects of incorrect application of:

1 Bleaches   4 Relaxer
2 Tints   5 Colour stripper
3 Perm lotion

To do

- Collect as many cuttings of hair in good and poor condition as you can find in your salon.
- Stick them down on paper and caption each with possible reasons for the condition.

Abnormal hair and scalp conditions

These may be:

- **Non-infectious** – they cannot be spread from one client to another, for example alopecia (baldness).
- **Infectious** – they can be spread from one client to another, for example head lice.

Non-infectious hair and scalp conditions

Although a non-infectious or non-contagious disorder may be unsightly, it is not catching and can be treated safely in the salon.

Infectious hair and scalp conditions

Infectious or contagious disorders **must not be treated in the salon**.

Deal with the client sympathetically and tactfully. Explain that you have found a certain hair or scalp condition which means that you cannot continue with their hair service. You must then recommend them to seek medical advice from either a doctor or a trichologist (a specialist in hair and scalp disorders).

All equipment must be cleaned and sterilised after contact with an infectious condition (see Chapter 6).

Non-infectious diseases and conditions of the hair and scalp

Name	Description	Causes	Treatment
Pityriasis capitis (dandruff)	Small, itchy, dry scales, white or grey coloured.	Overactive production and shedding of epidermal cells. Stress-related.	Anti-dandruff shampoos. Oil conditioners or conditioning creams applied to the scalp.
Seborrhoea (greasiness)	Excessive oil on the scalp or skin.	Overactive sebaceous gland.	Shampoos for greasy hair. Spirit lotions.
Eczema (sometimes called dermatitis)	Red, inflamed skin which can develop into splitting and weeping areas. It is often irritated, sore and painful.	Either a physical irritation or an allergic reaction.	Medical treatment.
Psoriasis (silver scaling patches)	Thick, raised, dry, silvery scales often found behind the ears	Overactive production and shedding of the epidermal cells. Possibly passed on in families, recurring in times of stress.	Medical treatment. Coal tar shampoo.
Alopecia areata (round bald patches)	Bald patches.	Shock or stress. Hereditary (i.e. passed on in families)	Medical treatment. High frequency treatment.
Male-pattern baldness (baldness, thinning hair)	Receding hairline, thinning hair. Baldness.	Genetic or hereditary.	Medical treatment is being developed.
Cicatrical (scarring) alopecia	A permanent bald patch where the hair follicles have been destroyed.	A scar from skin damage caused by chemicals, heat or cut.	None.
Sebaceous cyst (lump on scalp)	A lump either on top of or just underneath the scalp.	Blockage of the sebaceous gland.	Medical treatment.
Fragilitis crinium (split ends)	Split, dry roughened hair ends.	Harsh physical or chemical damage.	Cutting and reconditioning treatments.
Damaged cuticle (tangled hair)	Cuticle scales roughened and damaged, dull hair.	Harsh physical or chemical damage.	Reconditioning treatments. Restructurants.
Trichorrhexis nodosa (swollen, broken hair shaft)	Hair roughened and swollen along the hair shaft, sometimes broken off.	Harsh use of chemicals, (e.g. perm rubbers fastened too tightly during perming). Physical damage (e.g. from elastic bands).	Restructurants. Recondition and cut hair where possible.
Monilethrix (beaded hair shaft)	Beaded hair (a very rare condition).	Uneven production of keratin in the follicle.	Treat this hair very gently within the salon.

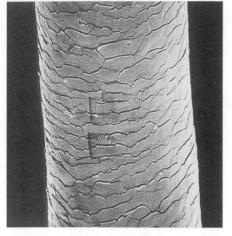

Smooth cuticles

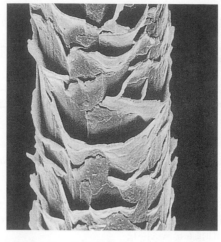

Damaged cuticles

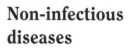
Non-infectious diseases

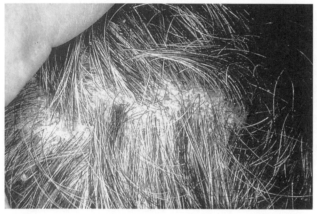

Psoriasis

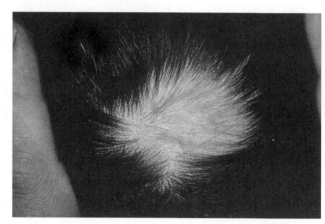

Alopecia areata

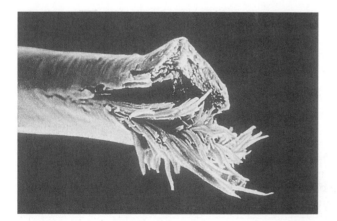

Fragilitis crinium

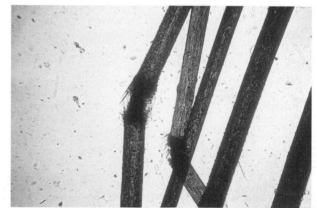

Trichorrhexis nodosa

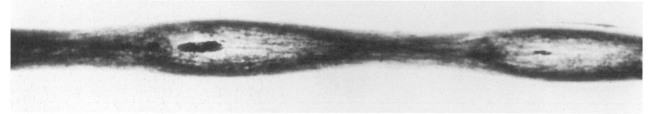

Monilethrix

Infectious diseases and conditions of the hair and scalp

Name	Description	Cause
Pediculosis capitis (headlice)	Highly infectious Small, grey parasites with six legs, 2 mm ($\frac{1}{12}$ in.) long which bite the scalp and suck blood. The female insects lay eggs called 'nits', which are cemented to the hair. Very common in children.	Infestation of headlice which lay eggs, producing more lice, living off human blood.
Scabies	An itchy rash found in the folds of the skin. Reddish spots and burrows (greyish lines) under the skin.	A tiny animal mite which burrows through the skin to lay its eggs.
Tinea capitis (ringworm)	Highly infectious. Pink patches on the scalp, develops into a round, grey scaly area with broken hairs. Most common in children.	Fungus. Spread by direct contact (touching) or indirectly through brushes, combs or towels.
Impetigo (oozing pustules)	Highly infectious. Blisters on the skin which 'weep' then dry to form a yellow crust.	Bacteria entering through broken or cut skin.
Folliculitis (small yellow pustules with hair in centre)	Small yellow pustules with hair in centre.	Bacteria from scratching or by contact with an infected person.
Warts (small raised lumps)	Small flesh-coloured raised lumps of skin.	Virus. Spread by direct contact. Only infectious when damaged.

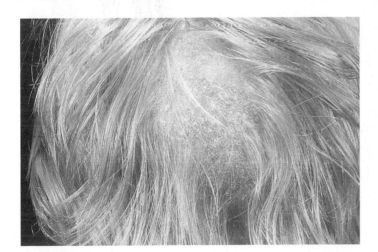

Tinea capitis (ringworm)

Infectious diseases

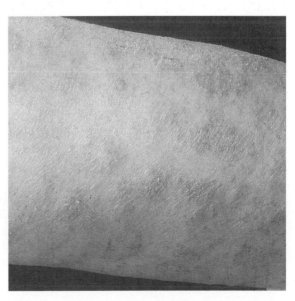

Scabies

Infectious diseases (Contd.)

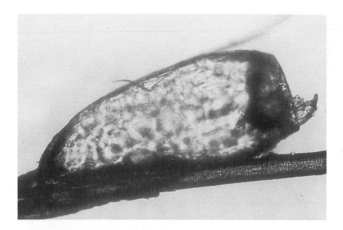

Pediculosis capitis (eggs or 'nits')

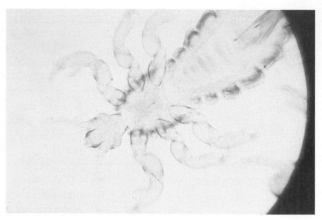

Pediculosis capitis

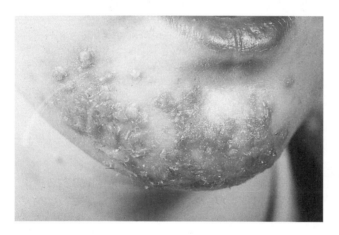

Impetigo

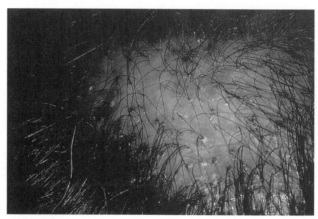

Folliculitis

Test your knowledge

1 Without looking at this book, describe each **infectious** and **non-infectious** condition and its cause.
2 List which **hair and scalp conditions** can be treated safely in the salon.
3 Describe the **treatments** available for conditions that can be treated in the salon.
4 List the conditions that **must be treated by a doctor**.

Designing a hairstyle to suit your client

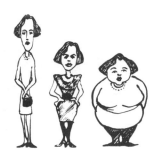

Have you ever wondered why two clients with exactly the same colour, texture and length of hair and the same hairstyle look quite different?

It is not only because of their height and build but also because of their head, face or neck shape. Clients must be advised according to these limitations.

Head shape

The shape of a person's head can be clearly seen when the hair is wet and combed flat against the scalp. For instance, if the head is flat on the crown you can compensate for this by leaving the hair longer in that area during cutting.

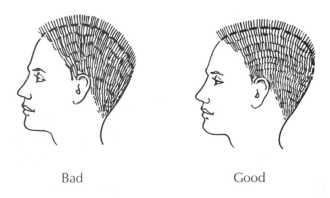

Bad   Good

Head shapes for a 'flat top' hairstyle

Head shapes can also be made to look quite different from the front just by altering the parting from side to centre. A side parting will make the head appear broader and wider, while a centre parting will make it look narrower and thinner.

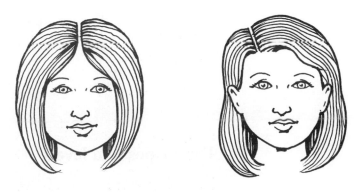

Centre and side partings

Face shapes

There are four main face shapes: oval, round, square and oblong (long).

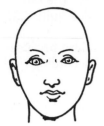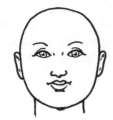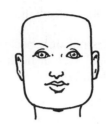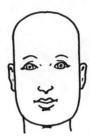

Oval

An oval face shape is ideal and suits any hairstyle.

Round

Round faces need height to reduce the width of the face. A straight centre parting will also help to reduce the width.

Square

Square-shaped faces need round shapes with wisps of hair on the face to soften them and give the illusion of being oval.

Oblong

Long faces suit short, wider hairstyles dressed around the sides of the face. A low side parting will also make the face look wider.

To do

■ Comb all your hair away from your face when it is wet and try to decide on your own face shape.
■ Make notes on your consultation sheets of different clients' face shapes.

Neck shapes

Long and thin necks are more noticeable with short hairstyles, and so need longer hair around them. Short necks can be made to look longer by an upswept or flicked style.

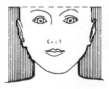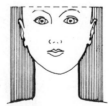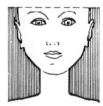

Ear shapes and levels

Generally, large ears, or even large lobes, are highlighted by hair cut short or dressed away from the face. It is better to leave the hair longer over the ears.

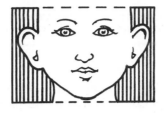
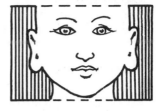
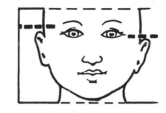

Large ears   Large lobes   Uneven ears

Some clients have ears that are uneven, so never balance a haircut by the level of the ears.

Nose shapes

A large nose will be more obvious from the side view when hair is drawn back from the face, whereas dressing the hair forward helps to minimise it.

Body build and height

One of the main reasons for consultation with the client before gowning up is so that you can briefly judge their body build and height.

Smaller clients can look overwhelmed by too much hair, or made to appear shorter from the back if their hair is too long.

On the other hand, large or overweight clients need a style with some volume and length to create a balance between their heads and their bodies. Short, flat hairstyles can highlight large bodies.

Age

A client's age is always an important consideration. Sometimes it is difficult to judge how old a person is, but generally softer styles with more movement are flattering for older people. Straight angular shapes are to be avoided.

Older clients also lose colour tone from their skin, so very few have naturally rosy cheeks; any redness is often caused by broken veins or cosmetic make-up. Dark or ashen colours can therefore be very ageing on older clients who, wishing to look younger, may want to return to the natural hair colour of their youth. Unfortunately this does not always suit them as they get older.

Client lifestyles

The client's lifestyle, occupation and personality are very important factors when choosing a hairstyle.

Lifestyle
The client could be a young working mother, who will not have much time to spend on her hair.

Occupation

Some occupations, for example the armed forces and catering professions, have strict rules about the length of hair.

Personality

A quiet, shy person may not be as daring with new styles as an outgoing extrovert. Clients are often worried about other people's reactions to a new hairstyle. A typical comment is: 'I'm not sure if my husband/wife will like it.'

Style books

Style books are very useful. They can be bought from hairdressing suppliers, or you can make your own. You can then adapt any of the ideas you have from the pictures to suit your **individual** clients.

To do

Make your own style book:

- Buy a plastic folder with clear plastic inserts to hold cut-out pictures of different styles.
- Illustrate the front cover with your salon's name and logo and **your name**.

You will need to include illustrations of **up-to-date fashion trends**, so try researching by:

- reading trade journals and magazines
- reading hair and fashion magazines and books
- watching television
- going to hair and fashion shows, hair seminars and trade exhibitions

Organise the style book in sections, e.g. short styles, long styles, styles to show hair colours, styles to show different types of perms, styles for special occasions (e.g. parties or weddings), and to suit different face shapes.

Test your knowledge

1 Describe how you can keep up to date with **current fashion ideas and trends**.
2 What type of **reading information** is available to help you keep up with changing fashions?

Hair growth patterns

Hair movement means the **amount of curl** or **wave already in the hair**, but **hair growth patterns** means the **direction in which the hair falls**.

This natural fall can best be seen on wet hair. If you comb your client's hair back from their face and gently push the head with the palm of the hand you can see the natural parting falling between the front hairline and the crown.

If you are cutting an all-one-length hairstyle such as a classic 'bob' then you must cut it to the natural parting. Otherwise, when the client tries to do their hair at home, the style could hang unevenly with long ends straying down.

There are several unusual hair growth patterns.

Double crown

If the hair is cut too short on the crown it is impossible for it to lie flat – the hair must be left longer.

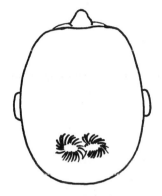

Double crown

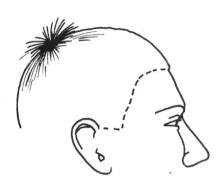

Unsuitable – crown cut too short

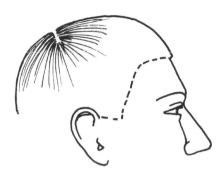

Suitable – longer crown hair

Cowlick

This is found at the front hairline and makes straight fringes on fine hair difficult to cut. It is better to sweep the hair to one side.

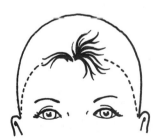

Cowlick

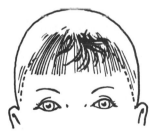

Unsuitable for full fringe

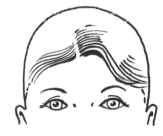

Suitable for uplift fringe

Nape whorl

This type of hair growth pattern makes straight hairlines difficult to achieve. It is better to cut the hair short into a 'V' shape or grow it longer so that the weight of the hair holds it down.

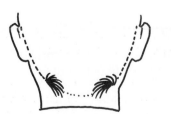

Nape whorl

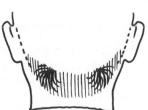

Unsuitable for short straight nape

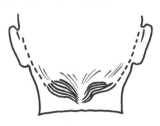

Suitable for 'V'-shape nape

Widow's peak

This is where the hairline grows forward at the front to form a strong centre peak. It is difficult to create a full fringe because the hair tends to separate and lift.

It is better to style the hair back off the face or create a very heavy fringe so that the weight of the hair helps the fringe to lie flat.

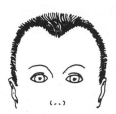 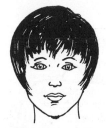

Test your knowledge

1 List the different types of **hair growth patterns**.
2 Describe how a **client's lifestyle** can affect your choice of hairstyle.
3 Name the **four main face shapes** and describe a suitable hairstyle for each.
4 Describe how hairstyling can correct **uneven head shapes**.

Explaining hair treatments to clients

Once you have decided on the type of hairstyle to suggest to your client you should explain it in simple terms. If you go into hospital for an operation, the doctor will explain what is going to happen to you in clear non-technical language to make you feel much more confident. You should do the same with your clients. Don't forget that some clients can feel quite anxious about certain hair treatments such as perming or colouring and may need reassurance.

If you explain a conditioning treatment as a 'cationic, deep-acting chemical which is substantive to the hair, penetrating deep into the cuticle layers and helping to reduce the hair's ability to absorb atmospheric moisture', the client may become somewhat confused!

However, if you say, 'I'd like to apply some of our own deep-acting conditioner to your hair to help the dry, flyaway ends become shinier and more manageable', the client will understand more about the product and why you are using it.

To do

■ Look up one method and procedure in this book for perming, colouring and bleaching. Write out a brief explanation of each in your own words.
■ Practise explaining the procedures to friends before talking to your clients.

Hair and skin tests

Whenever you are unsure about how a treatment will turn out you should test the hair first. Hairdressers always use a professional colour chart when selecting a colour so that they do not make mistakes. Testing helps to make both you and the client feel more confident.

Porosity test

Porous hair can absorb liquids (water or chemicals) through the cuticle and into the cortex.

If the cuticle is closed, flat and undamaged, the hair will feel smooth. However, once the hair has been physically or chemically damaged then it becomes generally more porous or unevenly porous. This is why special perm lotions are used for tinted and highlighted hair, as normal-strength lotions could quickly overprocess or hair colour could become patchy.

> **Remember**
>
> All hair is porous and can absorb liquids but over-porous hair or unevenly porous hair is difficult to work with and needs special care.

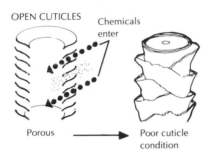
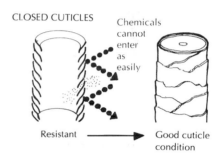

OPEN CUTICLES — Chemicals enter — Porous → Poor cuticle condition

CLOSED CUTICLES — Chemicals cannot enter as easily — Resistant → Good cuticle condition

Porous and resistant hair

Method
To carry out a porosity test, take a few strands of hair and hold them firmly in one hand near the points or ends and slide your fingers along the hair towards the roots. The rougher the hair feels the more porous it is, and the more damaged are the cuticle scales.

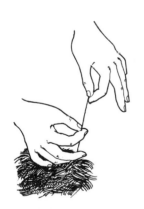

Porosity testing

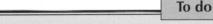

To do
■ Practise the porosity test on different types of hair.

Elasticity test

Well-conditioned hair is springy and bouncy; this means it has good **elasticity**. It can stretch up to one-third of its length when dry, half of its length when wet, and then return to its original length.

However, hair that has lost its elasticity because the internal chemical links and bonds in the cortex have been damaged may stretch up to two-thirds of its length or even break off.

Method
To test hair for elasticity, take some dampened hair between your thumb and forefinger and gently pull. If it stretches more than half its length then it is over-elastic and may break off.

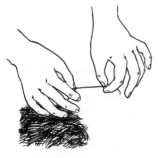

Elasticity testing

25

Incompatibility test

Some products that clients may have used on their hair may react badly with some of the chemicals that you intend to use – the hair may go green, steam or break off.

The most common products are **hair colour restorers**, such as Grecian 2000. They contain metallic salts such as lead acetate and the colour develops over a period of time. The hair often looks slightly greenish and feels harsh to the touch. The problem is that most clients do not admit to using them because **they do not consider they are colouring their hair** (they think they are restoring their natural hair colour).

In the salon a client with hair colour restorer on their hair **must not have**:

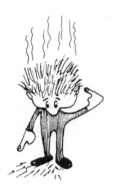

- a tint
- a bleach or highlights
- a perm (it is the perm neutraliser that reacts)

because all of these products contain hydrogen peroxide.

If you suspect a client has hair restorer on their hair, carry out an incompatibility test. Some temporary hair colours (colours that wash out of the hair), e.g. glitter sprays, also contain metallic salts and need to be removed.

Method

Mix 40 ml of 20 vol. (6%) hydrogen peroxide with 2 ml of ammonia (perm lotion will do) in a glass measuring container. Cut a few hair samples (use hair affected by metallic salts) from an unnoticeable area of the client's head and secure them with either cotton or sticky tape. Place the hair samples in the solution and keep them under observation. Results could take anything from 1 to 30 minutes to show.

If the hair has **changed colour**, if **bubbles have formed** in the solution or if the solution has **become warm** then there are definitely metallic salts on the hair.

Do not proceed with any hairdressing process that involves using hydrogen peroxide.

> **Remember**
>
> Always wear protective rubber gloves when you are using hairdressing chemicals.

> **To do**
>
> - Visit several chemist's shops and make your own list of all the products available that are similar to Grecian 2000 so that you can remember their names.
> - Practise an incompatibility test when the opportunity arises.

Colour test: taking a test cutting

In the same way that you would take a hair cutting for an incompatibility test from an unnoticeable part of the hair, you can easily test hair to see how it will take a hair colour.

Once the hair cutting is secured by cotton or sticky tape at the ends it can be tested with any of the following:

- Temporary colours – coloured setting lotions or coloured mousses.
- Semi-permanent colours – colour which lasts four to twelve washes.
- Permanent colours – tints that are mixed with hydrogen peroxide.
- Bleaches – used for highlights or general lightening.

Method

Mix a small amount of your intended product in a tint bowl and make sure that the test cutting is completely covered with it. Read the manufacturer's instructions to check the development time, but remember that the tints and bleaches will need longer than this to develop, because there is no warmth from the head to make them work.

After the development time, rinse off the semi-permanent, tint or bleach products (temporary colours are left on) and dry the test cutting. With the client, examine it under natural light (near a window) and decide whether both of you are happy with the result.

Test cuttings are also useful to show whether the hair will take the colour evenly, especially if it is unevenly porous.

To do

- Take test cuttings from white, blonde, medium-brown and dark hair and try them out with samples of your salon products.
- Attach them to cards and record all the details.

Strand test

A strand test is taken while the following products are on the hair to check when the product has developed thoroughly:

- Semi-permanent colours
- Permanent colours (tints)
- Bleaches
- Colour strippers (colour reducers)
- Relaxers

Method

Remove some of the product from a strand of hair with a piece of cotton wool or the back of a comb so that you can see whether it has developed properly, leaving the hair either the correct colour or the correct degree of straightness.

Pre-perm test curl

This test is taken if the hairdresser is in any doubt about the likelihood of a perm being successful. If the hair is in poor condition (over-porous or over-elastic) it is better to try out a few curlers first, rather than ruining the client's hair.

Method

Either cut a small piece of hair and tie it with cotton or proceed with a small section of hair on the head. Choose the strength of perm lotion and the appropriate size of rollers to use. Wind the hair around the roller, apply the lotion, develop it for the recommended time, then rinse and neutralise.

If the test is carried out on a hair cutting, once the curl is dry it can either be stored away or shown to the client immediately.

Pre-perm test curls are used to:

- Decide the **correct strength of perm lotion** to use
- Decide the **correct size of perm curler** to use
- Determine **how long** the perm lotion should stay on the hair (development time)
- Decide **whether the hair is in good enough condition** to take a perm – if in doubt, take an elasticity test.

Development test curl

This test is taken when the perm lotion is on the hair during the development process. Once the curl is fully developed the hair is neutralised.

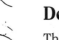

Unwind 1½ turns

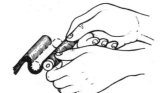

'S' shape to size of curler

Taking a development test curl

Method

Undo the rubber fastener from one end of the curler. Unwind the curler 1½ turns, without letting the hair unravel completely. Hold the hair firmly, with both thumbs touching the curler.

- **Using alkaline P/W lotions:** Push the hair towards the scalp, allowing it to relax into an 'S' shape. Do not pull the hair – remember it is in a very fragile state. When the size of the 'S' shape corresponds to the size of the curler, the processing can be stopped.
- **Using acid P/W lotions:** Push the hair towards the scalp and when it is developed it will separate into strands. This is called **stranding**.

> **Remember**
>
> Always check the manufacturer's instructions. Different perm lotions are checked by making different observations.

Test your knowledge

State how, when and why each of the following tests should be carried out:

1 Pre-perm test curl 　　　 5 Elasticity test
2 Development test curl 　 6 Incompatibility test
3 Test cutting 　　　　　　 7 Strand test
4 Porosity test

Describe the consequences of *not* carrying out each test.

> **Remember**
>
> **Para dyes** are toxic (**poisonous**) and can cause **allergic reactions** such as contact dermatitis (eczema) where the skin is red, swollen, itching and sore.

Skin tests

Many people suffer from allergic reactions to food or products (e.g. make-up). Hairdressing is no exception, and clients can become allergic to some hair colours. Permanent colours (which are tints mixed with hydrogen peroxide) and any semi-permanent colours containing **para dyes** always need a skin test.

To do
■ Check the instructions on all the types of colours in your salon to see which ones need a skin test.

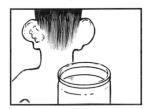

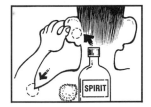

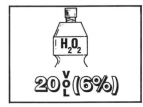

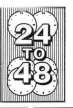

Skin tests must be carried out before each application of the hair colour (usually between 24 and 48 hours before). If the client has a positive reaction (redness, blistering, itching, etc.) para dyes **must not, under any circumstances, be used**.

Method

1 Clean a small, sensitive area of the skin (either behind the ear or in the crook of the elbow) with cotton wool and surgical spirit.
2 Mix a small amount of the colour to be used with equal parts of hydrogen peroxide, either 20 vol. (6%) or 30 vol. (9%).
3 Apply a small smear of the colour (about the size of a 20 pence piece) to the cleansed area. Allow to dry naturally.
4 Cover with collodian (New-Skin) and allow to dry.
5 Ask the client to leave the skin test for 24–48 hours, unless there is any irritation, in which case it should be washed off and calamine lotion applied to soothe the skin.
6 Record which colour and which strength of peroxide you used on a record card, together with the client's name, address and the date.

Check the skin test when your client returns to the salon. A **positive reaction** (redness, soreness, itching or swelling) means that your client is allergic to the colour. A **negative reaction** (the skin appears quite normal when the colour is washed off) means that you can proceed with the colour.

Test your knowledge
1 When and how should a skin test be done?
2 State the functions of skin tests in predicting reactions.
3 Describe the visible signs of a positive reaction to a skin test.
4 State the significance of a positive reaction.
5 State the significance of a negative reaction.
6 What could happen if a skin test was not carried out?

Consultation checklists

Once you have read this chapter and understood the variations in client's appearances and hair and scalp conditions you may find the checklists on pages 30–33 helpful.

Consultation and Diagnosis for All Salon Services

To be used for Unit/Element No. _____   Formative/Summative

Date _____   Hairdresser's name _____   Client's name _____

Client requirements

When was the client's hair last shampooed?   _____

Scalp condition   Dry/flakey/normal/oily (circle as appropriate)

Possible disorder/disease   _____

Hair   Texture   Coarse/medium/fine

Volume   Thick/medium/thin

Type   Afro/Caucasian/Asian

Movement   Straight/wavy/tight-curly

Look   Commercial/fantasy/avant-garde

Condition   Normal/naturally dry/resistant

Previous Chemical Treatments   P/W/relaxed/tint/ highlights/lowlights

Hair growth patterns   Nape whorl/widow's peak/cow's lick/double crown

Testing procedures   Elasticity/porosity/incompatibility/strand test/
Pre-perm test/skin test

Present style   V. long/long/medium/short/v. short
Layered/graduated/one length

Club cut/razored/clippered/other

_____

Consultation and Diagnosis for All Salon Services (Contd.)

Client requirements (Contd.)

    Client limitations   _____

    Any additional medical notes   _____

    Client lifestyle, personality, appearance   _____

    Client wishes   _____

    Suggested style   _____

    Shampoo/surface conditioner recommended   _____

    Time taken   _____

Conditioning

    Name of disorder   _____

    Product recommended   _____

    Massage movements   _____

    Equipment used   _____

    Time taken   _____

Cutting

    With/without fringe   With/without parting   Layered/graduated/one length

    Club cut/thinned/razored/clippered/other   _____

    Time taken   _____

Styling

    Thermal styling (Afro hair)   Full head/partial head/tonging/pressing

    Tools used   _____

    Finger dry/natural dry/blow dry

    Set description   Conventional/alternative

        _____

    Roller sizes   _____

    Pin curls   _____

    Styling products   _____

    Finishing products   _____

    Time taken   _____

Consultation and Diagnosis for All Salon Services (Contd.)

Chemical treatments

Perming	Virgin hair/tinted/bleached
Pre-condition	Yes/No
If yes, which product?	_____
Winding method	Root movement/uniform/non-uniform
Lotion type and strength	_____
Processing time	_____
With/without heat	
Time taken	_____

Neutraliser

Type	_____
Method	_____
Conditioning Products	_____
Time taken	_____

Relaxing

Corrective/virgin/regrowth/remove curl/reduce degree of curl

Product	_____
Method	_____
Processing time	_____
Time taken	_____

Colouring

Natural hair colour depth	_____
% of white	_____

Temporary/semi-permanent/quasi-permanent/permanent/bleaching/lightening

Full head/partial head/lighter/darker/highlight/lowlight

Product name and shade no.	_____

Consultation and Diagnosis for All Salon Services (Contd.)

Colouring (Contd.)

Peroxide strength _____

Method of application Conventional/alternative _____

Development time _____

Conditioning products _____

Time taken _____

Client statement

Did the stylist discuss your requirements
with you before any services began? _____

What advice have you received for
your hair and scalp care? _____

Did the stylist recommend products? _____

Would you have this stylist do your hair again? _____

Will you continue to follow the
recommendations? _____

Stylist signature _____

Client signature _____

Assessor signature _____

Test your knowledge
When you are using a consultation checklist why must you always identify any limiting factors regarding: ■ your client?   ■ the service being given?   ■ the products you will be using?

Selling skills

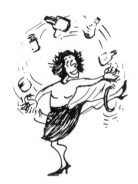

A salon exists for one reason: **to make money**. Staff need to encourage clients to visit the salon and keep visiting regularly. The most successful salons are those with **large, regular clienteles**. There is no better advertisement than a **satisfied client** with a **well-styled head of healthy looking hair**. A successful hairdresser must have:

- A regular **clientele**
- A good **personality**
- A strong sense of **professionalism**
- Good **expertise**
- The ability to **sell themselves** to their clients

What to sell

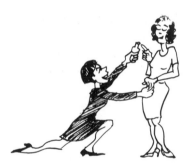

Hairdressers not only sell

- **products** – e.g. shampoos, conditioners, spray, mousse, gels, wax, etc. which enables the client to **maintain the finished style**
- **equipment and accessories** – e.g. combs, brushes, jewellery, hair ornaments, hairdriers, diffusers, tongs, etc.

but also advise about:

- the **salon**
- **themselves** (as stylists)
- **salon services and treatments**.

Therefore all staff must have a **full knowledge** of the services offered.

If you are worried about chatting to your clients, try to ask questions that are open-ended, such as 'How long have you been coming to this salon?' or 'How do you manage your hair when you go on holiday?' These cannot be answered simply by 'yes' or 'no', and help to get the conversation going.

Remember
Never discuss religion, politics, sex or race with clients, as you can easily cause offence and find yourself in an argument.

Try to develop a **sense of tact**. Bad atmospheres can often be created by a slip of the tongue, e.g. 'My goodness, you do have bad dandruff!' **Discretion** is also important. If one of your clients suffered from headlice, for instance, the worst thing you could do would be to tell other clients. Not only would these other clients worry that they might catch headlice, but gossip soon spreads and people might become wary of coming to your salon.

Try to increase your **general knowledge** by reading newspapers or by listening to news programmes on the radio. Once your confidence is established when dealing with clients, you can start to develop your selling skills.

To do

1 Open questions begin with 'How...?', 'What...', Which...?' etc.

Give some examples:

'How _____?'
'What _____?'
'Which _____?'
'Why _____?'
'When _____?'

2 Closed questions result in a simple 'Yes' or 'No' answer.

Give some examples:

'Do _____?'
'Have _____?'

Explaining various salon services

All the services that are available in your salon will be displayed on the price list. Clients will often ask about the benefits of different services. Here are some explanations you might give:

- 'Our reconditioning treatments work particularly well because we give a special massage to help them to penetrate into the hair.'
- 'We give two types of permanent waves. One is for a firm curl, the other is an acid perm which is gentler on the hair and will not dry it out.'

Here is a fuller description of a client discussion:

Discovering client needs
Stylist: 'Your hair has some pretty lightness at the very ends. Is that from your holiday last summer?'

Client: 'Yes, the sun lightened it, but it has nearly grown out now.'

Stylist: 'We could always place some natural-looking highlights through your hair to keep it going until next summer.'

Describing features of service
Client: 'Oh yes, how is that done?'

Stylist: 'By using either cap highlights or foil. The cap method is quicker and less expensive, but the foil gives more highlights exactly where you want them, and you can vary the colour.'

Client: 'What sort of colour would you suggest?'

Looking for buying signals
Stylist (uses shade cards): 'These light beige blonde tones exactly match the ends of your hair and would look very natural.'

Client: 'How long do they last?'

Describing benefits to client

Stylist: 'They will grow out gradually, and they give your hair a lot more body, which would help your fine hair to keep its style longer.'

Client: 'How much would they cost?'

Close sale

Stylist: 'They are normally £45.00 but we have a special offer for £35.00 if you can make a Monday or Tuesday appointment.'

Client: 'Yes, thank you, I'll make an appointment for next week.'

You can also use style books and product leaflets, rather than just words, to show the client what you mean. Clients will naturally want to know the cost of the service, so make sure you work it out correctly.

It is also important to explain to the client the **length of time** that different services will take. A short cut and blow-dry with little hair removed may take only 30–45 minutes, whereas a re-style, cut and blow-dry for a client with long hair which needs to be cut short may take well over an hour.

Retailing in the salon

All hairdressers have an excellent opportunity for selling products in the salon, in that they know **what to use** and **how to use it**. Once you have tried your particular salon mousse, for instance, you will understand its benefits (firm hold, non-sticky, gives lift, etc.) and find it easy to explain these benefits to your clients.

Remember

Some salon services include the cut and blow-dry, e.g. cut, blow-dry and perm for £45.00, while other services may not, e.g. conditioning treatments. These will also vary from salon to salon. Make sure that all staff know what is included in each of your advertised prices

---

To do

Make a short list of each of the products sold in your salon. Make a note of:

■ The benefits of each (e.g. normal hold, conditions dry hair)
■ How to use it (e.g. apply to towel-dried hair, apply with your fingertips)
■ The difference between similar products (e.g. conditioners for permed, coloured or naturally dry hair)

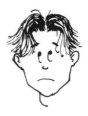

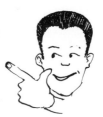

You can show the products to clients by the display at the reception area, but allowing clients to handle products also helps to sell them. If you allow the client to touch, feel or smell the product – especially when you are using it on their hair – you will always gain their interest.

Understanding your market

You will be selling hairdressing services and hairdressing products to many different **types of client**, each having different characteristics – long face, round face, high hairline, etc. This makes it important for you to recommend the correct product, service and hairstyle for each one.

Here is an example of how to sell a product.

Describe client needs
Stylist: 'Your hair is still a little dry at the ends; would you like me to use our new conditioner today, at no extra charge?'

Client: 'Yes please. What is this one?'

Describe product
Stylist: 'Well, it's one that you actually leave in the hair and don't rinse out. So it does save time.'

Client: 'Won't it leave my hair feeling sticky?'

Stylist: 'Not at all. Try a little on your hands. You can rub it into your skin and see it disappear. It works like that on your hair.'

Client (tries the product on her hands): 'Yes, my hands do feel soft and smooth.'

Describe features
Stylist: 'You can use it every time you shampoo your hair and also use it as a hand cream.'

Client: 'How much do I need to use?'

Describe how to use it
Stylist: 'Just squeeze out the size of a small coin, rub the palms of your hands together and smooth the conditioner into the ends of your hair.'

Client: 'Can I buy it at reception?'

Close sale
Stylist: 'Yes, the prices of all the sizes are clearly marked. Remember you get a hair conditioner and a hand cream for the same price!'

Once you have gained some product knowledge, you will find the best way to talk about it is in this order:

1 **Describe the product** – what it is (e.g. shampoo, hairspray).
2 **Describe how it works** – what it does (e.g. especially benefits permed hair or hair that is washed frequently, or prevents salon colours from fading).
3 **Describe how to use it** – e.g. hold the hairspray 30 cm away from your hair, or shake the can immediately before use.

Remember

- Whilst you are selling, use **the client's name** (it's the sweetest sound they know!)

- Learn to recognise **non-verbal** clues:

  Dilated pupils
  = 'I approve'

  Ear rubbing
  – 'I've had enough'

Use your common sense when selling services and products. For example, a
young working mother with no time to spare would be more likely to buy
a combined shampoo and conditioner or a 'wash 'n' wear' perm than a
senior citizen with more time on her hands.

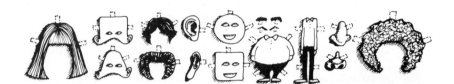

Selling: the three stages

The process of selling can be broken down into three stages:

1 **Finding out the client's needs**. This means identifying any previous
  treatments or problems. You will have learned to do this tactfully during
  the consultation process. Examples might include fine, lank hair, itchy
  scaly scalp, dry, split ends, etc.

2 **Giving the client advice**. This means asking any relevant questions that
  will lead you to suggest a particular service or product. Here are some
  examples:

- Fine, lank hair – 'Have you ever thought about having a soft body perm which just gives volume and bounce?'
- Itchy, dry scalp – 'Do you find your itchy scalp becomes worse with certain shampoos?' ('We have one which is especially soothing,' etc.)
- Dry, split ends – 'How often do you have your hair trimmed? We recommend cutting every six weeks to reduce split ends.'

3 **Gaining agreement with the client**. This is achieved by either receiving an immediate response or giving them time to think about it. For example, 'Would you like a perm on your hair now?' or 'My hair has been easy to manage with this perm. I'm sure that yours would be too.'

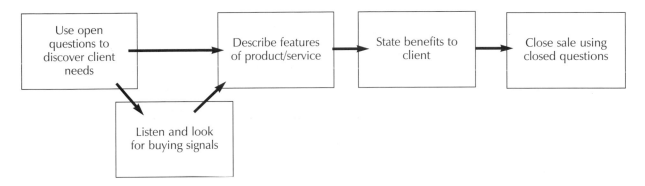

Finally, don't forget to record any sales or client services on your record card for next time.

Bad selling

If you were wondering where you went wrong, here are some common faults:

- Doing all the talking
- Knowing nothing about the product
- Interrupting – but not letting the clients interrupt you, thereby losing an opportunity for giving extra information
- Not listening, not 'hearing' unspoken thoughts, arguing
- Hard selling – working to a script, insisting the client buys the product
- Threatening – 'You won't get it cheaper anywhere else'
- 'Knocking the opposition', i.e. criticising other salons
- Manipulating – 'Oh dear, you'll make me miss my sales target'
- Treating 'No thanks' as a personal rejection
- Blinding clients with science
- Staying mainly silent, waiting for an order

Test your knowledge

1 Describe the five principles used during selling in the salon.
2 Using the list of client types on page 38, describe both suitable and unsuitable technical services, after-care products and equipment usage (if applicable) for each.

To do

- Read Chapter 14, page 212, on problems that can arise in the salon. Describe how you would cope with a client waiting for an appointment.

Client feedback

Client feedback should always be encouraged. It will help to improve your service and win repeat business.

It may be done in several ways:

- By using open-ended questions to obtain feedback from **both your own clients** and from **the clients of your colleagues**.
- By using **client questionnaires** (see Chapter 14, page 215).
- By having a **suggestion box** or a **client comment box.**

Whichever method you use, the feedback must be **reported** and **passed on**, so that it can be used constructively in the future.

To do

- Draw up a 'Lines of Communication' chart for your salon, stating each person's name, roles and responsibilities.
- Describe how your salon deals with client feedback. For example, is it through staff meetings, reports from the manager or open discussion?

Positive and negative feedback

Hopefully, most client feedback will be positive, but when **negative feedback** occurs, it must be dealt with in a professional manner. If a client approaches you with a complaint:

- Pleasantly and politely ask the client to sit with you in a **quiet area** of the salon so that you can discuss it in private.
- **Talk through the problem together** to diagnose the fault. When the complaint has been explained, **repeat it back** and confirm with the client that you have heard it correctly.
- **Don't argue with the client** – they will become more angry and create a disturbance in the salon. Stay calm, polite and understanding, never show your emotions. **Try not to take it personally.**
- **Diagnose the fault** and **suggest corrective action.**
- If the client agrees with your suggestions, then **carry out the correction** there and then, or agree a convenient return appointment.
- Always **record the complaint** and the action taken, and **thank the client** for bringing the problem to your attention.

To do

- Ask a friend to pretend to be a difficult client with a just complaint about their hair. Ask another hairdresser to watch and comment on how you deal with the situation.

Body language

Always take a deep breath and put on your **most sympathetic** face when faced with an angry client.

- Don't fold your arms – it looks too defensive.
- Don't lean too far forward – it may look aggressive.
- Don't make body contact – and keep a reasonable physical distance from the client.
- Don't clench your teeth, or tense your muscles – it may look as if you are trying to control your temper.
- Look interested and don't interrupt!

Serious complaints

If the client's hair is breaking off or they have a sore, inflamed scalp and you have not taken the necessary precautions, then:

- Never admit liability
- Consult with a senior member of staff or the manager

The senior member of staff or the manager must then:

- Notify the salon's insurers immediately that there is the possibility of a claim arising
- Pass on all correspondence unanswered to the insurers

It the worst comes to the worst and the situation is not resolved to the client's satisfaction, then the next call could be from the client's solicitor, or from the news desk of a tabloid newspaper.

Always pass media calls to the manager or owner.

Remember that client record cards and completed consultation sheets which include lifestyle questions and medical treatments may be a good defence in a court of law.

Prevention is better than cure! If your professional opinion is that you should not do the client's hair, then suggest something like 'Another hairdresser may well do your hair, but I'd like you to be a regular client and I'd like you to leave our salon feeling happy, so please be guided by my experience.'

Test your knowledge

1 Describe **three different ways** that you could **obtain feedback** from your clients on your salon's services.
2 Describe your **initial response** if a client approaches you with a complaint.
3 In the event of a serious complaint, what is the **next step** in the complaints procedure?
4 Why is it important to understand your salon's **lines of communication** when dealing with negative feedback?

2 Creative cutting

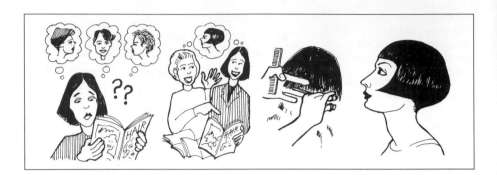

Designing a hairstyle

When choosing a hairstyle, hairdressers will usually work under three broad categories:

- **Classic** – i.e. the more timeless styles such as bob shapes
- **Fashion** – those that are currently 'in vogue'
- **Emerging fashion** – the forerunners of fashion

A hairstyle should be designed to suit each individual client and a good stylist should be able to adapt a style to suit any client.

To do

■ Put together a portfolio of classic, fashion and emerging fashion styles.

Many factors may influence your choice of style. These include:

- **Client personality, lifestyle and dress.** A client who is sporty or has a hectic lifestyle will need a style which is easy to manage and requires minimum styling.
- **Age of client.** Never assume that an older client will want an old-fashioned hairstyle.
- **Body shape and size.** The chosen style must be in proportion with the body.
- **Face shape and features.** The style should be designed to suit the face shape and enhance, or disguise, facial features.

To do

■ List the four main face shapes and think of some features:
  - that may need disguising
  - that should be emphasised.

Client consultation

Carrying out a **thorough** consultation with the client before commencing, using style books if desired, will give both the stylist and the client a clear picture of what is to be done.

Checking with the client as the cut progresses is also a good idea as this allows any necessary adjustments or changes to be made. Consulting with your client before and during the cutting process will help to prevent any problems from arising and promote a professional image of the salon. It will also help to ensure **client satisfaction**. If clients feel that you have not only produced a good result but have also been attentive, listened to their concerns and given good advice, they will be encouraged to return to the salon and may even promote the salon and its services to their friends.

HEALTH MATTERS

Remember to check hair and scalp for any contagious disorders during your consultation. Failure to recognise potential infections or infestations could result in infecting yourself and others (cross-infection).

To do

■ Re-read Chapter 1 on Client Care and giving advice.

The hair

As well as client limitations, the hair itself must be considered before deciding on a style. Each of the following will influence the style and cutting techniques chosen:

● **Thickness/density**
● **Texture**
● **Length** – short, medium, long
● **Condition and quality** – remember to carry out porosity and elasticity tests
● **Hair type** – European, Afro-Caribbean, Asian
● **Hair growth patterns** – cow's lick, nape whorl, widow's peak
● **Existing body or curl** – curly, wavy, straight

To do

■ Give examples of how each of the factors listed above could influence cutting and styling.

By paying attention to these influencing factors you will be able to create a hairstyle which will **maximise the potential** of the client's hair, producing the best possible result and creating a style which not only suits the client but also **complements** their lifestyle, appearance and personality. Ways of enhancing the hair cut include the addition of colour and perming services. Colouring techniques can be used to enhance the look of the haircut, for example a semi/quasi colour can be applied to give shine and gloss to a sleek bob or slices/strands of hair can be coloured to give definition and emphasise particular areas of a haircut. Some styles may need additional curl, body or root movement, which can be provided by perming, in order to recreate a specific look or to make the style easier for the client to manage at home.

To do

■ List the cutting services offered in your salon and how much time is allocated to each when booking appointments.

Preparation of client

Always gown up the client using a cutting gown which totally covers their clothing so as to protect it from water and hair cuttings. In many salons a cutting collar is used in place of a towel to keep the neck free from obstruction when cutting. When using clippers a strip of cotton wool can be put under the neck of the gown to catch any hair clippings

Preparation of tools and equipment

Make sure that all cutting tools and equipment are clean and sterilised before use and that equipment is positioned for ease of use but is out of the reach of any children in the salon. When using electric clippers always make a visual check of cables, plugs and switches before use and remember to turn off the power supply after use.

Health and safety when cutting

Health and safety are very important when cutting hair. When handling cutting tools, avoid accidents by:

- **Never** carrying cutting tools in pockets
- **Taking care** when replacing and using open-blade razors
- Keeping cutting tools **in protective cases** when not in use
- Keeping sharp tools **out of the reach of children**
- Learning how to use each piece of cutting equipment **correctly**
- **Cleaning and sterilising** equipment after use
- **Storing safely** in an allocated area

To do

■ Find out your salon and local authority procedures for the disposal of used razor blades (sharps) and why it is important to dispose of them correctly.

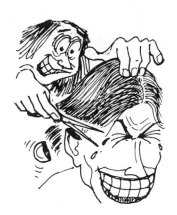

Accidents when cutting

Accidentally cutting the client
If an accident does happen, **keep calm** and give the client a **sterile dressing**, asking them to apply this to the cut with pressure to stop bleeding. Do not touch the cut yourself because of health risks such as AIDS and Hepatitis B. Small cuts may be covered with a sterile dressing but larger cuts may need medical attention.

Accidentally cutting yourself
Many hairdressers cut themselves during hair cutting. **Stop** whatever you are doing and excuse yourself from the client. **Rinse the cut with water** to remove any hairs, then apply pressure with a **sterile dressing** until the blood clots and bleeding stops. Dry the area and apply a sterile plaster.

Cleaning cutting equipment

Metal cutting tools can be cleaned by wiping with cotton wool and **surgical spirit** to disinfect them. They can also be sterilised in an **ultraviolet cabinet**. Liquid disinfectants are not advisable as prolonged use can cause the metal to become corroded. An **autoclave** can also be used.

The cut

Because cutting is a creative process it is not possible to have rules for every haircut. Stylists develop their own style of working, but each haircut must be **controlled**.

The cut is controlled by:

- **Accurate guidelines.** The first cut in each section **determines the length** for the rest of the section. Guidelines must be followed for an even haircut.
- **Correct angles of hair to the head.** Many angles may be used when cutting the hair. They will affect the **shape and balance** of the cut.
- **Correct angle of cut.** Many angles can be used, depending on the chosen style. They will also affect the shape, balance and length of the hairstyle.
- **Clean and neat sectioning.** This will make sure no meshes are missed and that you work in a **neat, methodical way,** which gives a more professional appearance and result.

Baselines

Many hairstyles have clearly defined **perimeter**, or **outer**, design lines. Within these design lines the hair may be **one length**, **graduated** or **layered** and a variety of lengths. Many styles are based on variations of the following design lines. Different effects can be created depending on:

- The **angle** they are used in relation to the head
- The **combination** of one or more lines
- The **type, texture and density** of the hair

Straight baseline
Hair is cut to a horizontal line, producing an even result (below left).

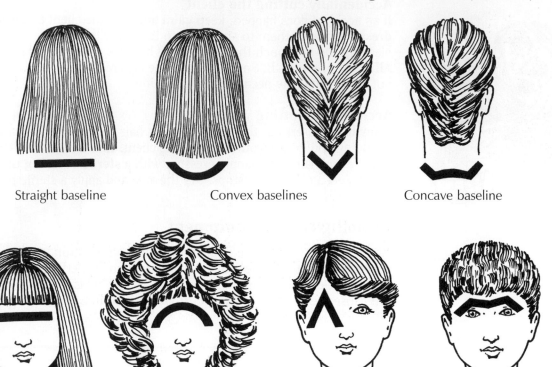

Straight baseline   Convex baselines   Concave baseline

Fringing and layering

Convex baseline
Hair is cut so that the **centre back section** is cut **longer** than the sides (above centre). A steep angle will encourage hair to fall **from the shortest point to the longest point**, whereas a **soft curve** will produce a '**U' shape** if used at the nape.

Concave baselines
The hair is cut so that the **centre back section** is **shorter** than the sides (above right). An **inverted 'V'** will push hair away from its central, shortest point, whereas a **soft curve,** when used **at the nape of the neck**, will give a straight line – this is often used to give an even result when cutting hair with a **nape whorl**.

These lines can also be used when cutting fringes or when layering the hair to produce different results (when fashion styling).

Layering

There are many different forms of layering. Listed below are the most popular methods.

1. Basic layer
The basic layer method produces layers that are of an even length throughout the head by holding sections at a 90° angle from the head throughout the hair cut.

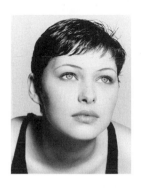

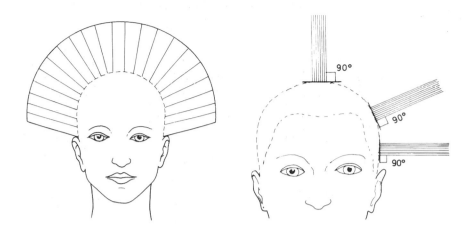

2. High/increase layering

Sometimes called **high graduation**, this method produces shorter layers through the **top and crown area**, becoming longer through the **back and sides**. This is achieved by holding top sections at 90° and increasing this to 180° as you progress to the back and side sections by **over-directing** (pulling hair upwards) to meet the shorter layers. See colour plate 1.

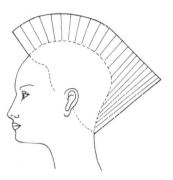

3. Graduation

This method gives a style in which the **inner layers** are **longer** than the **outline shape**. Once a guideline has been cut (usually at the hairline), sections are held at 45° from the head, either vertically or horizontally, and cut to create graduation. See colour plates 1–2.

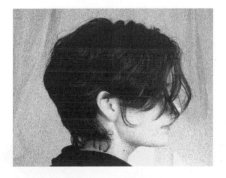

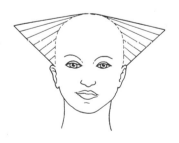

4. Reverse graduation

Used when cutting hair to one length. Once the initial guideline has been cut, each subsequent section is cut slightly longer, allowing the hair to turn under easily. This technique is often used when cutting a bob.

Cutting techniques using scissors

Club cutting

This is the most common cutting technique. However, it must be precise and is often called **precision cutting**. The sub-section of hair must be cleanly combed through and held with an even tension before cutting.

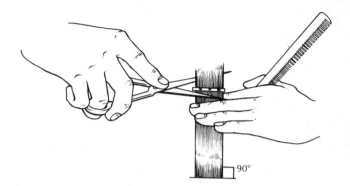

The diagram shows hair cut at 90° for a layer cut, but the hair may be cut at any angle to the head according to the style planned. Club cutting may be done on wet or dry hair and the ends of the hair are left blunt and heavy (this is sometimes also called **blunt cutting**).

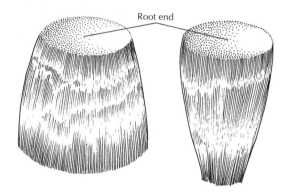

Root end

Taper cutting

Taper, **slither** or **feather** cutting will reduce both the length and the thickness of the hair. This technique is done on dry hair and, unlike club cutting, the hair is cut underneath the fingers.

Tapering is a sliding, slithering, backwards-and-forwards movement along a sub-section of hair. Close the scissor blades as you move towards the roots.

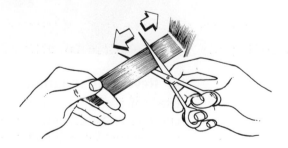

Freehand cutting

This is where the hair is cut **without being held in place** with tension from any forced directional pull. The hair is combed from its section and allowed to fall into its own natural movement before cutting.

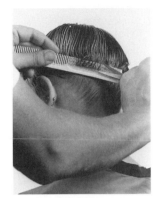

- It is a particularly useful technique during one-length cutting, where a straight line is required. On below shoulder-length hair, holding the hair with a finger underneath can cause unwanted graduation.
- Cutting fringes with a cowlick will naturally make the hair bounce up too short if it is cut with tension.

Scissor over comb

This technique is used to give the **same effect** as **'clipper over comb'** work. The hair around the nape and sides is cut short, following the contours of the head.

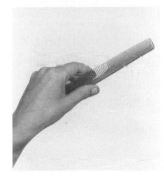

Use a cutting comb to pick up the hair, keeping the scissors parallel to the comb during cutting. Use the comb in an upwards direction, lifting the hair so that the hair sticking through it can be cut off. Move the comb and scissors continually towards the top of the head, keeping the comb up and out and away from the head, cutting at the same time.

Thinning hair with thinning scissors

These scissors remove only **thickness** or **bulk** from the hair, **not length**. They are sometimes called **aesculaps**, **serrated** or **texturising scissors**.

Ordinary thinning scissors can be used to thin out from the middle of the hair, cutting diagonally across the sub-section of the hair. Open and close them two or three times to remove the thickness.

Many new variations on the normal thinning scissors have now been developed, and the different shaped blades can be used to create a variety of exciting effects.

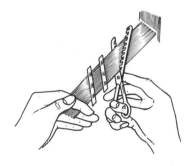

Cutting techniques using clippers and razors

Clippers

Electric clippers are now commonly used for both men's and women's hairdressing to give the same effect as the 'scissor over comb' technique.

Clippers have two blades with sharp-edged teeth. One blade remains fixed while the other moves across it. The action of the motorised moving blade is similar to several pairs of scissors being used at the same time, which is why many hairdressers like the speed of cutting with clippers.

Detachable clipper heads are available so that the closeness of the cut can be altered. The **larger** the number, the **longer** the length; the **smaller** the number, the **shorter** the length.

Razors/hair shapers

These can be used to create fashion styles and are ideal for creating soft, wispy outlines and textured styles.

The two main types of razor in use are:

- **Open** or **cut-throat** razors
- **Shapers** or **safety** razors

Both are used on wet hair because razoring on dry hair is painful for the client. Razors must be kept sharp or they will tear the hair.

Open or cut-throat razors

Open razors may be used to **shorten** the hair and to **remove thickness**. They are used underneath or above the wet sub-sections of hair and are stroked towards the ends with a scooping movement that produces a tapered effect. Many hairdressers also use open razors to create a clean hairline around the haircut.

It is important to **hold a razor safely** so that it does not close up on your hand during cutting. Open razors are now available with **disposable blades**. These are more hygienic, and as one blade becomes blunt you can replace it, so you always have a sharp edge to use.

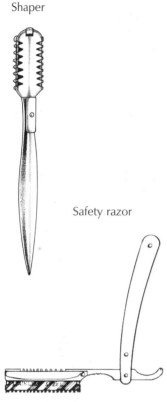

Shaper

Safety razor

HEALTH MATTERS

Always use a new razor blade for each client if the blade is to come in contact with skin and dispose of in a sharps container or wrap carefully in cotton wool and paper and secure before placing in a bin.

Shapers or safety razors

These razors have a guard over the blade so that only part of the hair is cut. They produce a **feathered**, **uneven** effect and are easier and safer to use than open razors.

Combining cutting techniques

Fashion styles are created by combining a variety of basic cutting techniques to produce the desired result. Personalising the cut using texturising techniques gives an individual look.

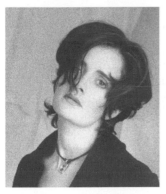

Combined cutting techniques

Texturising techniques

Listed below are some examples of texturising techniques.

Twist cutting

Twist small sections of hair and either chip into section using points of scissors or use tapering action to remove hair.

Slicing

When the outline shape of the haircut is achieved, comb the hair into style, slightly open the blades of the scissors and position on the section of hair to be sliced, then slide blades down the section to remove hair. This technique is best used when texturising front hairlines, fringes and sides.

Pointing and texturising

Pointing can be used to achieve **feathered effects** and to **soften hard lines** created by club cutting.

Take a sub-section of hair and insert the scissors over the fingers to chip out small pieces at the ends of the hair. When **larger pieces** are taken out of the hair, this is called **texturising**. See colour plates 3–4.

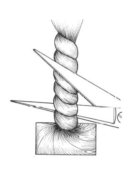

Twist cutting

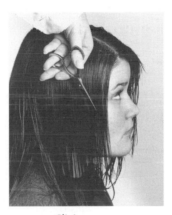

Slicing

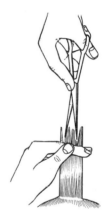

Point cutting

Weave cutting

Take a section of hair and weave, as for highlighting. Drop the hair you wish to leave longer and cut the remaining woven strands. The result can be either drastic or subtle depending on the size of the weave and the effect required. Thickly woven strands will produce a quite dramatic, severe result whilst fine strands will give a subtle result.

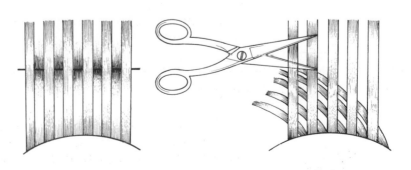

Finishing techniques

It is important not only to have the skills to carry out cutting techniques to produce a particular haircut but also to know which products, tools, equipment and techniques can be used to dry the hair into shape and create a finished result. This will enable you to advise the client on how to recreate the style her/himself.

To do

■ Find a selection of pictures that incorporate all the cutting techniques listed below and give a brief description of which cutting techniques and tools were used and what cutting angles, outline and internal shapes would be used to recreate the look. Also include details of styling and finishing techniques, products, tools and equipment used for each haircut.

- Tapering
- Thinning
- Freehand
- Texturising
- Scissor over comb
- Club cutting
- Layering
- Graduation
- Reverse graduation

Test your knowledge

1 Why should you pay attention to **influencing factors** when cutting hair?
2 Why should the **client's lifestyle** be considered when designing a hairstyle?
3 What **safety considerations** should you take into account when cutting hair, and why?
4 How should you **dispose** of hair cuttings?
5 Why is it important to **consult with the client** throughout the cutting process?
6 What is the best type of **scissors** to use when **slicing** the hair?
7 List the different **baselines** and the results produced by each.
8 List the different techniques of **layering** and the results produced by each.
9 When would you **texturise** the hair by **chipping/point cutting**?
10 Why is it important to ensure **client satisfaction**?
11 Describe what is meant by **classic**, **fashion** and **emerging** fashion styles.

3 Perming

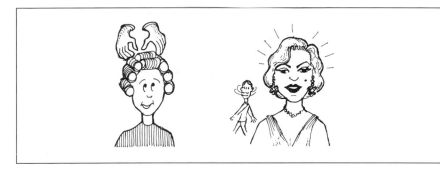

Clients today look for more in a perm than just curls. They require **volume**, **lift**, **body** and **texture**, all of which will give support to, and enhance, their hairstyle.

To do
■ Write a list of all the perming services provided by your salon and the time allocated for each.

Client consultation for perming

Remember
Small cuts or abrasions on the scalp can be protected using Vaseline or barrier cream.

A good perm depends not only on your practical skills but also on your ability to make the **right decisions** about your client's hair, both **before** and **during** perming. Prior to perming, carry out a thorough **hair and scalp analysis**, ensuring that there are no contra-indications, for example, infectious or contagious conditions, scalp abrasions or non-contagious disorders such as psoriasis. Make sure that the hair is in good enough condition to withstand a perm. Listed below are some points to help you when carrying out a consultation.

Cutting

Most hair will need cutting, either to remove any perm on the ends or to re-style before perming. Some hairdressers prefer to cut the hair before perming, others choose to cut after perming.

When using a perm for more **creative effects** or **adding body and volume** to the hair, it is advisable to cut the hair into style **before** you begin your wind, as this will allow you to see exactly where lift, texture and movement are needed within the hairstyle.

Finishing techniques

During consultation the stylist must establish how much time the client will spend on the upkeep of their new style and also how they will look after their new perm. Remember – soft, big curls, waves and volume will not last as long as a traditional perm and the client must be advised of this.

Very often a client will have a picture showing the look they wish to achieve, and in some cases the hair in these pictures has been styled after perming by setting or tonging. As hairdressers we must explain to the client what they would/will have to do to recreate the look they want or we have created for them. Take time during the consultation process to explain how the client can maintain their style at home using suitable shampoos and conditioners, styling and finishing products, tools and equipment.

To do

■ Look through some style magazines and consider the products, tools and equipment that would be needed in order to recreate various styles.

Perming tests

It is important to carry out diagnostic tests both **before** and **during** the perming process. This will help to ensure that the correct products, tools, equipment and winding techniques are used. It also minimises the possibility of any problems arising and ensures the best possible results.

To do

■ Re-read the sections in Chapter 1 on the following tests which are relevant to perming:

　– Pre-perm test curls
　– Elasticity tests
　– Porosity tests
　– Incompatibility tests
　– Development test curls

Note the purpose of each test and the method of carrying it out.

Perming coloured and bleached hair

Hair that has been permanently coloured or bleached is more porous and will absorb perm lotion very quickly. You must, therefore, choose a strength of lotion especially for this type of hair (often no. 2, 3 or 4 strength; you will need to **refer to the manufacturer's instructions**).

Some hair is unevenly porous (e.g. very dry ends) and will need a **pre-perm lotion** applied to those areas of hair to even out the porosity. Pre-perm lotions are applied to towel-dried hair and left on; they are **not rinsed out before perming**. Pre-perm lotions usually come in liquid form and have three functions:

● They even out the porosity of the hair, thus allowing the perm lotion to penetrate the hair evenly and process all parts of the hair at the same rate.

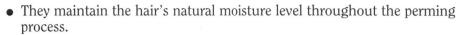

- They maintain the hair's natural moisture level throughout the perming process.
- They help to keep the hair damp, reducing the need to keep spraying the hair with water.

Some products also contain agents which can protect the client's scalp, preventing scalp irritation.

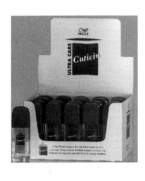

Some companies also produce **perm regulators**. This type of product usually comes in the form of a thick gel and is designed for use when carrying out any type of wind where **some sections** of hair **do not require perming** or on hair which **may already have curl** in the mid-lengths and ends and is in need of re-perming at the **root area only**. They work by restricting the amount of lotion that enters the cortex of the hair that the perm regulator has been applied to, allowing a small amount of lotion to penetrate but not enough to break any bonds.

The chemical process of perming

Understanding the chemical process of perming will help you to select the **correct type of lotion** for your client's hair.

There are three stages in perming:

1 **Softening** – The hair is softened by the perm lotion
2 **Moulding** – The lotion causes the hair to take up its new shape whilst it is wound around the perm rods
3 **Fixing** – The hair is fixed permanently using neutraliser

> **Remember**
>
> An 'S'-shaped curl movement should be formed when the processing stage of an alkaline perm is complete, and the hair will separate into strands on an acid perm. If you see a definite 'S' formation on an acid perm this shows that the hair is overprocessed.

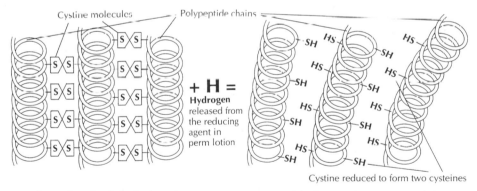

Cystine molecules   Polypeptide chains

+ **H** = **Hydrogen** released from the reducing agent in perm lotion

Cystine reduced to form two cysteines

Breaking the disulphide bonds   Hair moulded into shape around the perm rod

Softening and moulding the hair during perming

The strong disulphide bonds in the hair are made of an amino acid called **cystine**. These are the bonds that are broken by the perm lotion during the perming process. These bonds are broken because alkaline perm lotions contain a **reducing agent** called **ammonium thioglycollate** (you can smell the ammonia when you open the bottle).

Most perms will process **without** the use of **additional heat**. However, if the salon is cold, the processing time can be **speeded up** by using an **additional heat source** such as an **accelerator**. Always check the manufacturer's instructions to see if they recommend using additional heat.

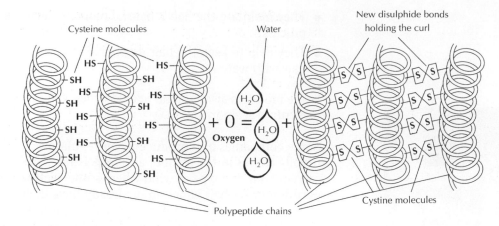

Disulphide bonds broken by perm lotion   Hair fixed in its new curled shape

As the perm lotion soaks through the cuticle scales and enters the cortex, the reducing agent adds hydrogen to the disulphide bonds, to form a new amino acid, **cysteine**. The hair is now softened and will mould itself to the shape of the perm rods. Once the correct degree of curl is achieved neutralising agents containing either hydrogen peroxide or sodium bromate, which produce oxygen, are applied to the rods in order to fix hair into its new position.

Neutralisers come in a variety of forms and concentrations. Some can be applied directly to the perm rods from an applicator bottle, others require dilution before application by sponge or in an applicator flask. Most neutralisers require a development period but some now available work instantly on contact with the hair. These products are often more beneficial when neutralising fashion winds.

Conditioning the hair after perming

Once neutralising is complete, applying an **anti-oxidant conditioner** to the hair will **replace moisture**, **close the cuticle**, **restore the hair** to its natural pH level and **prevent any neutraliser** that may remain in the hair **from continuing to oxidise** (sometimes known as **'creeping oxidation'**)

Choosing an acid or an alkaline perm

Alkaline perms

These have a pH of approximately 9.5, which opens up the cuticle scales, makes the hair more porous, and allows the perm lotion to enter the cortex.

The **higher** the perm lotion's pH, the **more damaging** it is to the hair. This is why conditioning agents are added to alkaline perms, and why acid perms are becoming increasingly popular.

Acid perms

These have **activators** added to them and generally rely on **heat** to open up the cuticle scales so that they can penetrate the cortex. The exception to this is when using an acid perm on **bleached hair**: as the cuticle layer is already damaged, additional heat may not be necessary. Remember: always check the manufacturer's instructions as products will vary. They generally have a slightly acid pH (5.5–7) and contain a chemical called **glyceryl monothioglycollate**.

Fewer bonds in the hair are broken by acid perms, which is why they are said to be better for use on damaged hair and hair that is easy to process.

> **Remember**
>
> Acid perms must be used immediately after mixing to ensure optimum results.

> **Remember**
>
> Acid perms are best suited to damaged, chemically treated, bleached or fragile hair.

Matching hair type to perm lotion

The choice of **lotion type** and **strength** is dependant upon the **hair and scalp analysis** and **test results**. Perm lotions are available for many different types of hair:

- **Resistant** – non-porous, fine hair which often dries very quickly, or some types of coarse white hair
- **Normal** – virgin hair that has not been treated with chemicals
- **Tinted** – hair that has been processed with permanent tints
- **Bleached** – hair that has been processed with bleach (including highlights)
- **Over-porous** – hair that is in a very dry, porous condition

Hair that is generally more porous needs a weaker perm lotion, and resistant hair needs a stronger perm lotion. **But whatever type of lotion is used always adhere to the manufacturer's instructions on suitability and use.**

After using products and materials for perming, always **update stock records** and **report any stock shortages** to the relevant person for action. Shortages of stock can lead to inability to carry out some perming services.

> **To do**
>
> ■ Briefly describe your salon's requirements for reporting stock shortages.

Preparation of client

It is best to gown up the client using a **dark-coloured gown** and disposable plastic cape as well as towels. In some cases, for example when carrying out a spiral wind, it is also advisable to use a drip tray to protect the client's clothes from chemicals. Barrier cream can also be applied to the client's skin around the hairline to help prevent any skin irritation.

Preparation of self

Always **wear gloves** when applying perm lotion to protect your hands from chemical damage and skin irritation.

Preparation of tools and equipment

Before you begin your wind, **have all the tools, equipment and products** necessary for you to complete the perm **on your trolley** or work station; this will ensure that everything is readily available and within easy reach, and will help you to work more efficiently. **Clean up** work areas and dispose of any waste as you go along to help **prevent accidents**, **minimise** the risk of **cross-infection** and help to promote a **professional image** of yourself and the salon to clients.

HEALTH MATTERS

Always check that all tools and equipment have been properly sterilised before using them on clients.

To do

■ List the three ways of sterilising equipment used in the salon.
■ Check the manufacturer's instructions and your salon policy for information on the safe disposal of chemical waste.

Winding techniques

The following are examples of current and emerging perm winds:

Spiral winding

This method of winding has become very popular over the past few years. Spirally winding the hair gives a uniform, even curl along the length of the hair and is suitable for long, one-length hair.

Tools
Conventional perm rods, Molton Browners (available in foam and rubber), tubes and chopsticks.

Method
Divide the hair from forehead to nape into two sections of equal size.

Long layered styles

PLATE 1

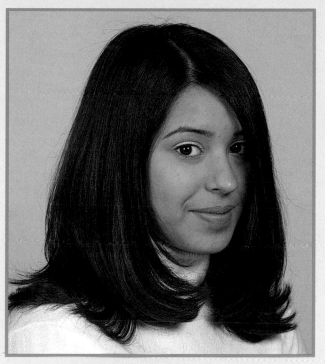

Style 1

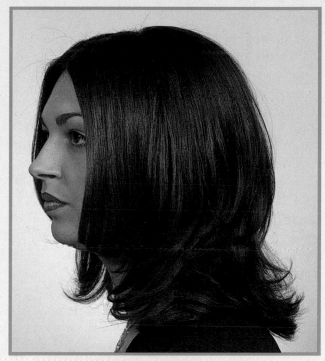

Style 2

Graduation variation step-by-step cut

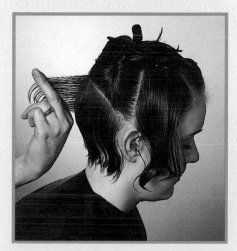

Step 1
Section above occipital bone. Starting at centre back, work parallel to head, cutting vertically into nape.

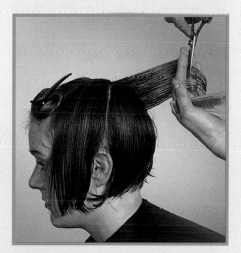

Step 2
Section from crown to top of ears. Continue working vertically, following guide from previous sections, working hair parallel to head.

PLATE 1

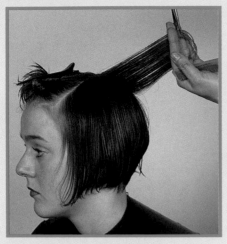

Step 3
Continue working through crown, lifting at 45° to create a gradual build-up of weight.

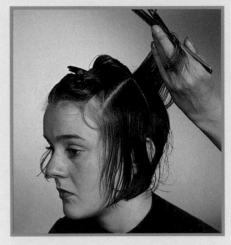

Step 4
Start working at same angle through side sections to front of ear.

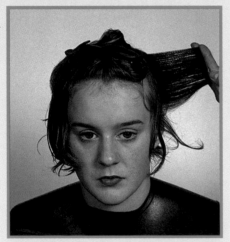

Step 5
Work with diagonal sections through sides and over direct back to maintain length and weight in front area. Repeat other side.

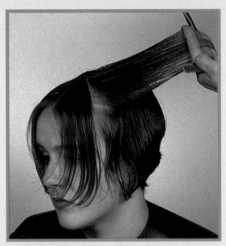

Step 6
Continue diagonal sections through to front area; blend remaining hair.

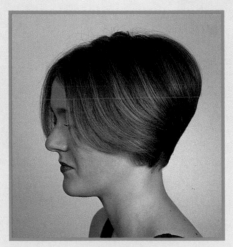

Step 7
Blow-dry with vent brush for smoothness and large round brush for fullness at crown.

PLATE 2

Textured layering step-by-step

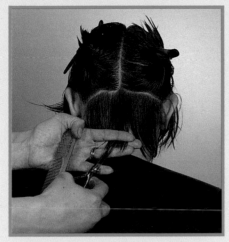

Step 1
Keeping length, texturise by cutting into each section about $\frac{3}{4}''$ deep. Keep control of hair to maintain balance.

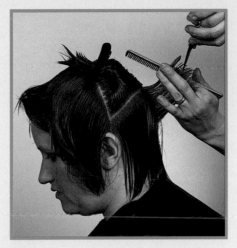

Step 2
Work technique through layering in the occipital bone area.

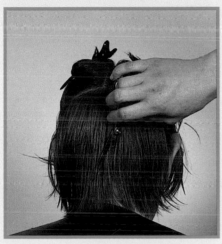

Step 3
When layering is complete, slice through hair to reduce weight.

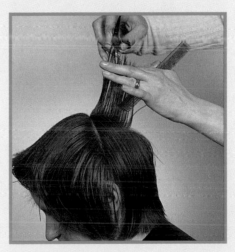

Step 4
Continue through crown, slicing hair to create a feathery effect.

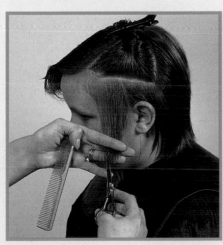

Step 5
Take a side section and using the same technique reduce weight and length.

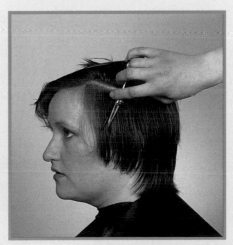

Step 6
Work as step 3. Repeat on other side.

PLATE 3

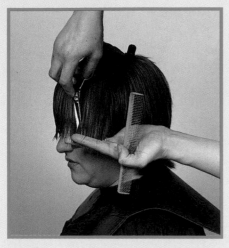

Step 7
Connect fringe with sides using same technique.

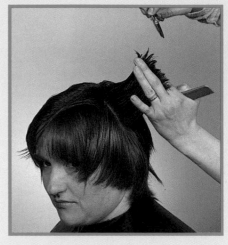

Step 8
Using guide from back, work textured layers through sides.

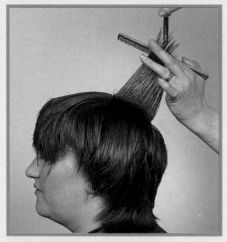

Step 9
Work same technique through crown.

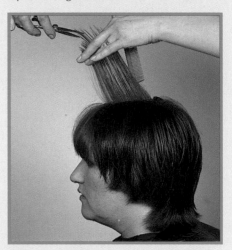

Step 10
Work layers through fringe area.

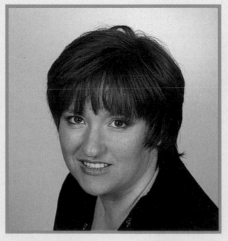

Step 11
Finger-dry back, smooth fringe with vent brush and use wax for definition.

PLATE 4

Perm winds

PLATE 5

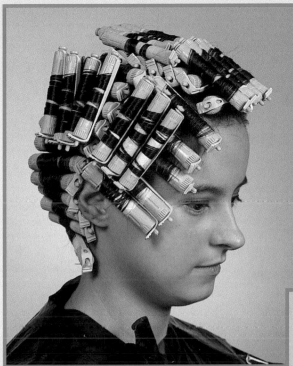

Hopscotch wind

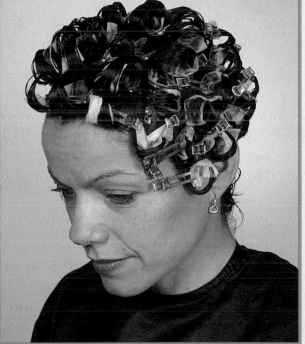

Pin curl wind

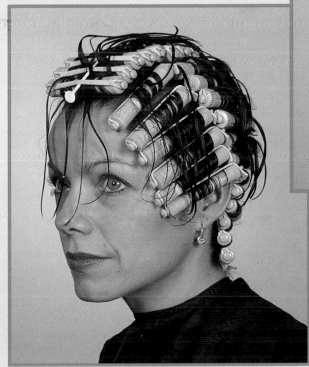

Weave wind

Random highlights step-by-step

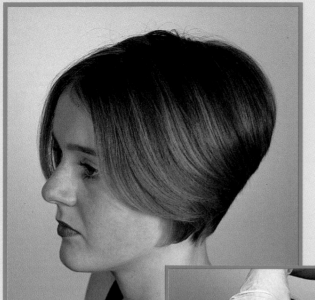

This technique is ideal for use on sleek, one-length hairstyles. The effect produced can be altered by taking larger sections to give a bolder result and using a variety of colour combinations.

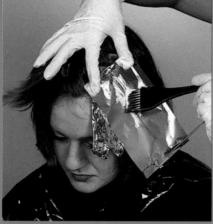

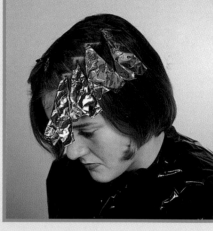

Step 1
Take zigzag section along scalp. Lift peak of inverted 'v' with pin-tail comb and separate from other hair. Place square of foil under hair strand and apply chosen colour.

Step 2
Fold foil into a triangle-shaped packet to secure and prevent slipping. Repeat along zigzag section, colouring the peaks only.

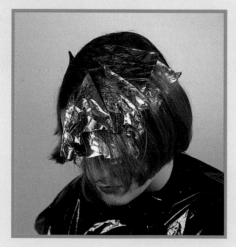

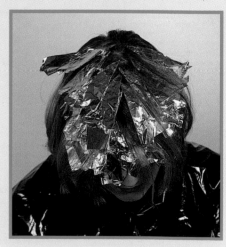

Step 3
Repeat the zigzag parting on next sections to be coloured and proceed as for steps 1 and 2.

Step 4
Once completed, develop colour until desired shade is achieved, remove by shampooing and style.

PLATE 6

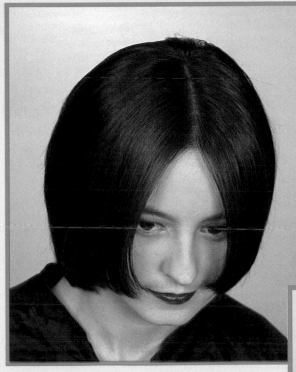

Block colouring

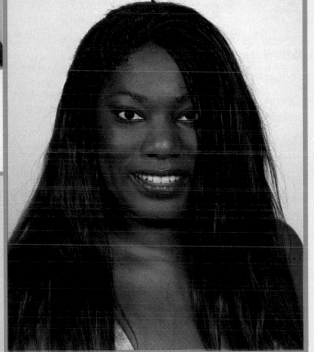

Hair extensions

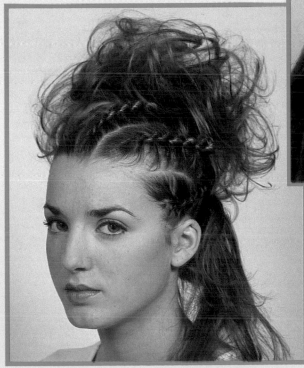

Alternative styling

PLATE 7

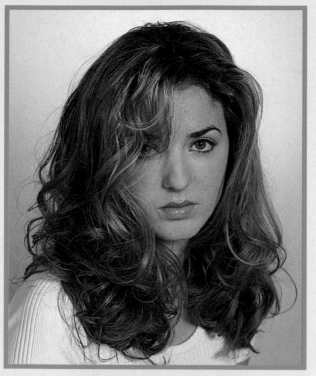

Curly style

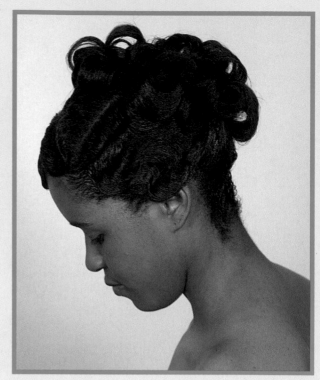

Classic styling

Twists and knots

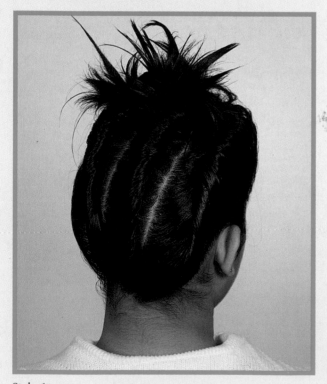

Style 1

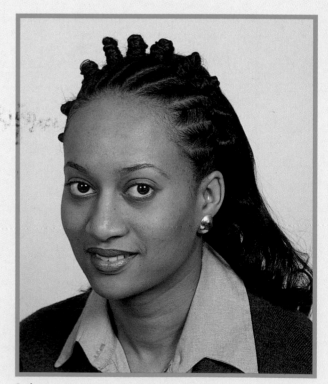

Style 2

PLATE 8

The depth and width of each section to be wound depends on the amount of curl required.

For best results and maximum curl, take sections between 1.25–2.5 cm ($\frac{1}{2}$–1 in.) deep.

The width of each sub-section will depend on the diameter of the rod used.

Method using Molton Browners (or equivalent)

Take a sub-section of hair and place end paper to cover ends of hair. Start winding from the bottom of the rod. Turn the rod, **spiralling the hair up along its length**. Once you reach the hair roots, bend the rod over to keep it in place.

Once this first row is completed, continue to take further sections, working up the head in the same way.

Tip: Wind hair around end paper several times to prevent hair unwinding.

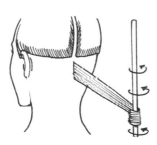

Spiral winding

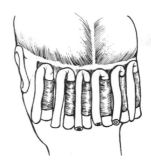

Spiral wind in position

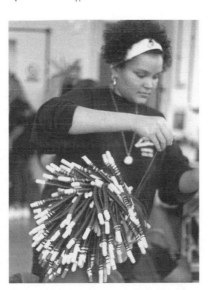

The rods in place

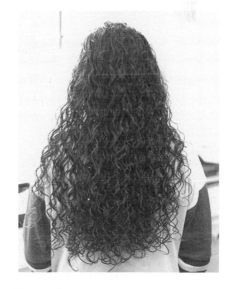

The result

Hopscotch wind

This method of winding gives the hair **texture**, **volume** and **varying curls**, producing a **non-uniform curl result**, and is suitable for one-length hair or hair with long layers (see colour plate 5).

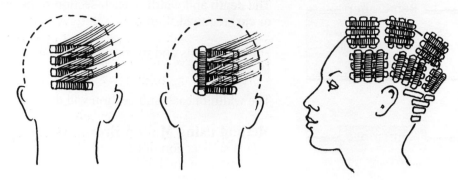

The hopscotch wind

Tools
Conventional perm rods, style formers (Wella), techniwavers (L'Oréal), rovalers (Wella).

Method
- Take a normal-sized section and **weave thickly**.
- Wind the **back half** of this section onto a rod.
- Continue in this manner until **four or five rods** have been wound, leaving unwound hair between each rod.
- Taking **vertical sections** of woven hair, wind so that the rod **sits vertically** on the previously wound section.
- Continue to wind all areas in the same way.

This wind can also be achieved simply by splitting a normal-sized section of hair and winding instead of weaving each section.

> **Remember**
>
> This wind can be used on a whole head or specific areas to create irregular curls.

Piggy back wind

This method will give the hair **texture**, **volume** and **varying curls**, producing a **non-uniform curl** result. It is suitable for one-length hair or hair with long layers.

Tools
Conventional perm rods, style formers (Wella), techniwavers (L'Oréal), rovalers (Wella).

Note: To create **varying curl strengths**, **different sizes**, or **types**, of rods can be used.

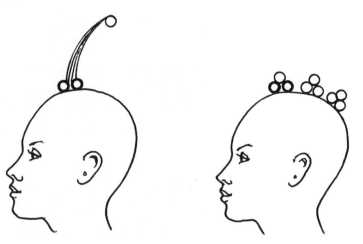

The piggy back wind

Method

- Take a fine section of hair and wind as for a **basic wind**.
- Take next section, but **do not wind**. Comb out of the way and leave.
- Take **third** section and wind as for first.
- Next, wind the **middle section**. This will sit on top of the **previously** wound rods.
- Continue to wind the remaining hair in the same manner.

This technique can be used on the whole head or in specific areas where extra volume is needed.

Note: Each section **must be fine**. If the sections taken are too thick, the centre rod will fall between the others and not sit on top.

Double/twin wind

This technique gives **varying curls along the hairs' length**, creating **looser movement** at the roots and **curl along lengths and ends** of hair.

Tools

Conventional perm rods work best.

Method

- Take section of hair and wind around rod.
- When half of the hair's length is wound, **add another rod** to the section and continue to wind both rods together down to the roots and secure.
- Continue to wind the rest of the head in the same manner.

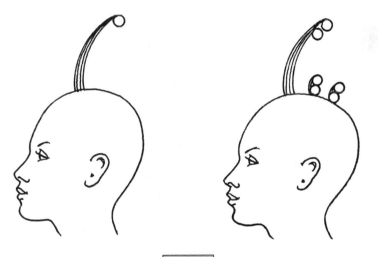

The double/twin wind

To do

- Ask your product manufacturers/suppliers for information on new innovations for root perming, etc.

The following techniques are best suited for use on **short hair**, creating volume rather than curl. Various manufacturers have developed products especially for the needs of this type of client – for example **Headlines** by **Wella**, which gives style support and enables the service to be carried out more frequently than a conventional perm.

Weave wind

Gives **root movement**, **volume** and **texture** to short hair (colour plate 5).

Rods
Conventional, style formers (Wella), techniwavers (L'Oréal).

Method
- Take a normal-sized section of hair and **weave thickly**.
- Wind the **back half** of this section onto a rod, **leaving the front part straight**.
- Continue until all areas to be permed have been wound.
- **Barrier cream** can be applied to the woven sections which are **not being permed** to protect the hair from perm lotion.

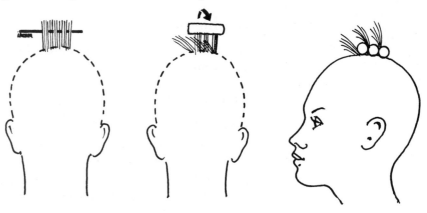

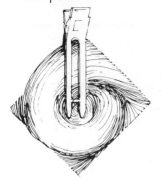

The weave wind

Pin curl perm

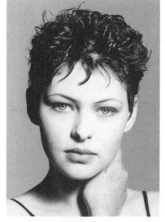

Pin curl perm

Gives the hair **root movement**, **volume** and **texture** (colour plate 5).

Tools
Lady Jane clips, either metal or plastic.

Method
As when setting hair using pin curls, sections can be **square**, **oblong** or **triangular**. **Stand-up barrel curls** will give **root lift** and **volume**, whereas **flat barrel curls** with a closed centre will give **stronger curl movement**.

Before starting, it is important to **plan your wind**, including the **direction of curls** and where **volume is required**, to ensure the desired result is achieved.

- Put end papers around hair points, form the hair into a pin curl and secure with a Lady Jane clip.
- **Cotton wool** can be put into **stand-up curls** to **prevent them collapsing** when lotion is applied.
- Continue to form curls on all areas of the head to be wound.
- A **hairnet** can be placed over the head during **neutralising** to **protect the curls**.

Barrelspring curl

To do
■ Cut pictures from style magazines and describe how you could re-create each look. Include a description of the tools and equipment, winding techniques and products you would use on different types and lengths of hair.

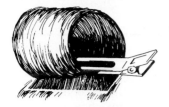

Stand-up barrel curl

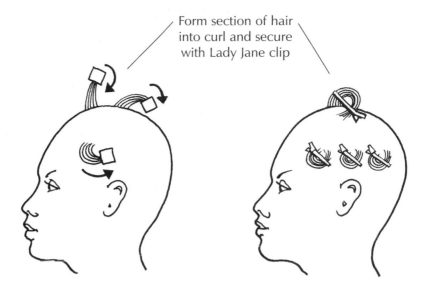

Form section of hair into curl and secure with Lady Jane clip

Safety points to remember

- Make sure that the **client is comfortable** throughout the service.
- Check that **perm rods** are **not causing discomfort** and that there is not **excessive tension** on rods (loosen off perm bands).
- Applying lotion can be very **dangerous**, as it can easily run into the client's eyes. If this does happen, **rinse immediately** with cold water on a pad of cotton wool until the stinging stops.
- Always use a strip of **dampened cotton wool** around the hairline and hold a piece of cotton wool during lotioning to use for absorbing any excess.
- **Pull burns** may result if the hair is wound tightly – the neck of the hair follicle opens, allowing perm lotion to enter. If the scalp is scratched, this irritation could become infected, causing **folliculitis**.
- Many manufacturers' bottles of perm lotion and neutraliser look very similar. To avoid applying the **wrong lotion**, do not take out the bottle of neutraliser until you are ready to neutralise.
- When rinsing the hair make sure that the **water temperature and flow are suitable** for the client at all times
- Familiarise yourself with manufacturers' instructions and your salon policy for the storage, use and disposal of perming and neutralising products. This is also covered under COSHH regulations 1992.

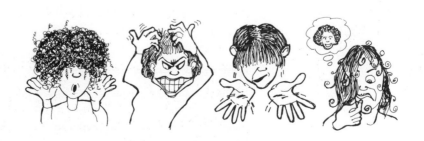

Perming faults and corrections

Fault	Causes	Correction
The perm is not curly enough (weak curl).	Poor shampooing (hair greasy). Poor neutralising. Perm rods too large. Too few perm rods used. Perm lotion too weak. Not enough perm lotion applied. Perm lotion not left on long enough. Incorrect angling and placing of perm rods.	Re-perm the hair using a weaker perm lotion, but clip the rest of the hair well away from the perm lotion.
Hair too curly.	Perm rods used were too small.	May be gently relaxed if condition allows.
Overprocessed hair (looks frizzy when wet and straight when dry).	Perm lotion too strong. Too much heat used during processing. Too much tension used. Rods too small.	Suggest a course of conditioning treatments and regular haircuts. Do not re-perm the hair: it will break off.
Scalp/skin damage or irritation.	Perm lotion or relaxers coming into contact with scalp/skin – if it enters the hair follicle, 'pull burns' occur. Barrier cream not applied to sensitive skin areas. Cuts and abrasions to the scalp.	Remove any excess perm lotion with water. Apply a soothing moisturising cream to the area.
Hair breakage.	Too much tension during winding. Rubber too tight or twisted. Perm lotion too strong. Hair overprocessed.	Suggest a course of reconditioning treatments or restructurants.
Band marks.	Rubbers placed wrongly on the hair. Too much tension.	Restructurant, deep-acting conditioner.
Deterioration of hair condition.	Overprocessing.	Restructurant, deep-acting conditioner.
Uneven result.	Incorrect sections. Uneven application of lotion and neutraliser. Uneven tension used.	Re-perm straight areas.

Client record cards

When you have completed your perm always complete a client record card, giving full details of any products, tools, equipment and winding techniques used. If your salon uses a computer to store client details, re-read the section in Chapter 1 which deals with the Data Protection Act.

To do

- Write a list of all the information that should be contained on a client record card.

Test your knowledge

1 Why is it important to carry out hair and skin tests **before** and **during** perming processes?
2 What **personal skills** should you use when giving advice to clients?
3 Why should you consider the **image** of the client when perming?
4 What **personal protective equipment** should be used during perming? Why?
5 Why is it important to record and report **stock shortages**?
6 List three methods of **sterilising** tools and equipment.
7 Why is it important to work **safely** and keep work areas **clean** and tidy?
8 Under COSHH regulations, how should you dispose of **chemical waste**?
9 List the common **perming faults** and how to correct them.
10 List and describe a range of **perming products** available for use.
11 List the **health and safety** points to consider when perming hair.

4 Colouring

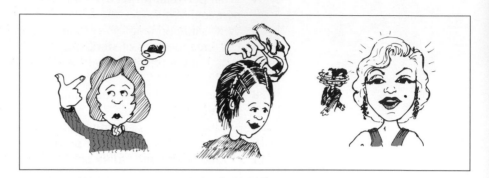

There are many reasons for a client to choose to colour their hair – to cover white hairs, enhance an existing hairstyle, or simply because they want a change of image.

Before you colour a client's hair, it is important to understand the effects of colouring products on the hair, how to choose a complementary colour, how to apply a variety of colouring techniques, and what to do if a problem occurs. The colouring services offered by you and your salon should not only be for the benefit of the client but should also enhance the salon's image. It is important that hairdressers keep up to date with new techniques and methods of colouring hair so that they can provide a variety of services and satisfy the needs of each individual client.

Preparing the client for colouring or bleaching

Gowning up

It is best to gown up the client with a plastic or rubberised bleaching or tinting gown to protect their clothes from any chemical splashes. Most salons also use towels, shoulder capes and tissues around the neck area.

If you are using very dark colours, or the client has sensitive skin, you may also need to use protective **barrier cream** around the hairline.

To do
■ List the procedures for gowning and protecting clients for colouring services in your salon.

Preparation of self

Always **wear gloves and apron** when using colouring or lightening products, to protect your hands from chemical damage and skin irritation and your clothes from staining or damage.

Preparation of tools and equipment

Before you begin colouring, check that you have sufficient products and materials needed to carry out the technique you have chosen. Position all the tools, equipment and products necessary for you to complete the colouring service on your trolley or work station – this will ensure that everything is within easy reach and will help you to work more efficiently. **Clean up** work areas and dispose of any waste as you go along to help **prevent accidents**, **minimise** the risk of **cross-infection** and promote a **professional image** to your clients. Once you have completed your work, update any stock records to prevent stock shortages, which may cause inconvenience to clients and disruptions in salon services.

> **To do**
>
> ■ Briefly describe your responsibilities for dealing with stock shortages.

Safety points to remember

- **Before** commencing any colouring services **check the manufacturer's instructions** and your salon policy for the safe storage, use and disposal of colouring products.
- **Carry out all necessary hair and skin tests.** If colouring product is to come in contact with the client's skin, look at the manufacturer's instructions to see if they recommend carrying out a skin test before use.
- **Always check** the client's scalp for any **inflammation**, **cuts** or **abrasions**. If you are in doubt whether to proceed, ask another stylist for a second opinion.
- **Clean up** any spillages immediately.
- Ensure that all **tools and equipment** are **properly sterilised** by using chemicals, such as disinfectant, heat (for example an autoclave) or an ultraviolet cabinet.
- If you chose to use an additional heat source to help speed up the colouring process, make sure it is designed to be used with colouring products. Also **check the equipment for electrical safety** before using.
- Make sure that the client is comfortable throughout the service.
- When rinsing the hair make sure that the water temperature and flow are suitable for the client at all times. Remember – the scalp can be sensitive to water temperature after colouring.
- Staying alert to possible hazards throughout the client's visit will reduce the risk of accidents.

> **Remember**
>
> If using an additional heat source bear in mind that too much heat can damage hair, particularly if using lightening products.

Hair texture and porosity

Check the hair texture and porosity. Remember that some coarse-textured hair can be resistant to colour and unevenly porous hair (dry ends) can absorb colour unevenly. Take a test cutting if you are unsure about the result.

> **To do**
>
> ■ List all of the hair and skin tests that should be carried out when colouring hair and describe why, when and how each of them should be carried out. What are the potential consequences of failing to do these tests?

Record cards

Quite a lot of information is needed when colouring and bleaching a client's hair, so always complete the record card straight away in case you forget any of the details. As many salons now use computers to store client information, these records are subject to regulation under the Data Protection Act. Re-read the section in Chapter 1 which details the principles of this act.

To do
■ Write a list of all the colouring services provided by your salon and the time allocated for each.

Points to remember when choosing a hair colour

Client's requirements

- How light or dark (**depth**) do they want the colour?
- What **tone** do they want, e.g. red, copper, ashen?
- Use the **shade chart** to decide together.

Manufacturers of colouring products are regulated by the International Colour Code system (ICC,) which identifies the depth and tone of colours on a colour chart.

To do
■ Refresh your memory by drawing and labelling a simple diagram of a colour star/circle.

Client's natural (base) colour

Very dark hair cannot be tinted to light blonde (you will have to pre-lighten with bleach).

Amount of white hair present

The more white hair present, the brighter any warm tones such as red and copper will show up.

Hair condition and porosity

Unevenly porous hair will absorb colours unevenly.

Hair texture and density

Some coarse-textured hair is resistant to colouring, so take a test cutting first.

Complexion and skin tones

Never colour an older client's hair too dark or too ash – it will make them look older.

To do
■ Re-read the sections in Chapter 1 on giving advice and guidance to clients.

Bleaching hair

Hairdressers use bleach to lighten hair when other products such as highlift tints are not strong enough.

Clients who have naturally 'mousy' hair that lightens in the sunlight may wish to recreate this effect by bleaching. Blonde hair is often considered to be more flattering, especially with sun-tanned skin, and once clients have experienced being blonde they often feel that their own colour is less exciting.

Blonde highlights are easier to sell to clients, especially on layered hair where the natural-coloured regrowth is less obvious. The initial cost of highlights, especially woven highlights (which take more time) may be high, but they need to be repeated only every few months. If clients prefer a full head bleach, then the regrowth must be done every few weeks.

Bleaching materials

Emulsion bleach

Emulsion bleaches are made up of three separate parts:

- An **oil** or **gel** bleach
- **Hydrogen peroxide** (normally 20 vol. [6%] or 30 vol. [9%])
- **Boosters** or **activators** (sachets of powder)

Always check the manufacturer's instructions for the recommended strength of peroxide and the number of boosters or activators to use.

Make sure you **mix up** in the **correct order**. The peroxide and boosters are generally mixed first and then the oil or gel bleach is added so that it does not become lumpy.

Emulsion bleaches are particularly good for **whole-head** and **regrowth** bleaches as the consistency makes them easy to apply and they are formulated to be gentle on the scalp.

To do
■ Look at the emulsion bleach left in the bowl after it has been used and see how much it has expanded due to the release of oxygen.

Powder bleach

Powder bleaches are made of two parts:

- Bleach powder
- Hydrogen peroxide (normally 20 vol. [6%] or 30 vol. [9%])

Powder bleaches have to be mixed to a smooth paste, but check the manufacturer's instructions as the **amount of peroxide** will vary if you are using **liquid**, as opposed to **cream**, peroxide.

Powder bleaches are also **strong bleaches** and are generally used for highlights and fashion effects. However, they have a tendency to **dry out** and become powdery if excessive heat is applied.

Always measure, check and mix bleach products carefully, **checking the manufacturer's instructions**. If you use peroxide that is **too strong**, or mixtures of bleach that are **too thick**, you could **burn** the client's scalp and give an **uneven colour** to the hair. Peroxide that is too **weak**, and bleach mixtures that are **too thin**, can run into the client's eyes, skin and clothes and will **not lighten the hair enough**.

The chemistry of bleaching

All bleaches are **alkaline** and contain **ammonia** (you can smell this quite strongly when mixing bleaches). The alkali in bleaches has two actions:

- It swells the hair and opens up the cuticle scales so that the bleach can enter the cortex and lighten the colour pigments.
- It mixes with the hydrogen peroxide and releases the oxygen, which will bleach out the colour.

Hair when bleached will always lighten in this order:

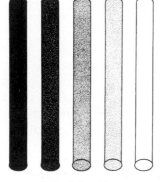

Peroxide effects

1 Black
2 Dark brown
3 Medium red brown
4 Light warm brown
5 Light golden brown
6 Medium golden blonde
7 Light blonde
8 Very light blonde
9 White (disintegration)

Hair must **never** be allowed to lighten beyond a very light blonde colour or it will disintegrate completely.

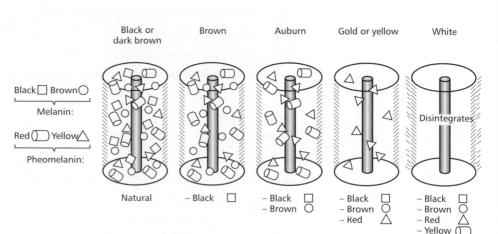

Bleaching out colour pigments

Application methods

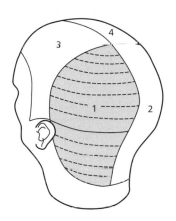

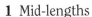

Hair may be lightened with **highlift tint** (mixed with special developers), **emulsion bleach** or **powder bleach**, depending on the client's **natural base shade** and the **degree of lift** required. Generally, dark hair will need the stronger bleach products to lift. If in doubt, take a test cutting.

Whole head

Both whole-head and regrowth bleaches are usually applied to hair sectioned into four as shown in the diagram on the left.

Bleach is usually applied to the nape or crown area first where the hair is more resistant. Always apply bleach to a whole head of virgin hair in this order:

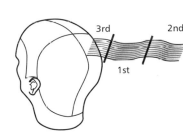

1 Mid-lengths
2 Ends of the hair
3 Roots of the hair

This is because the client's **body** heat (from the scalp) will make the bleach take **more quickly** near the scalp.

Never skimp with the amount of bleach. Take very small sections and always check the application thoroughly. The smallest area left uncovered will show up disastrously.

Regrowth application

When applying bleach to regrowth, always be thorough and **never overlap** on to the previously bleached hair, as hair breakage could occur.

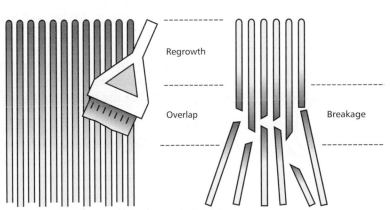

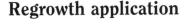

Hair breakage from overlapping

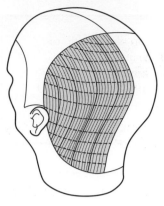

Cross-checking the application

Checking the application

You can never be too careful when applying bleach. Always check the application from the opposite direction to the one in which you applied it.

If you have missed any areas, apply bleach to them immediately, or dark patches will be seen. Pay special attention to the hairline and the thickest part of the hair (i.e. behind the ears).

Removing the bleach

Whole-head or regrowth bleach

Remove the bleach product by **rinsing thoroughly** until the water runs clear. Use a lower water temperature than usual because the client's scalp will be sensitive, but ask the client if the temperature is comfortable.

Then **gently shampoo** the hair. If a bleach toner is to be used then do not use a conditioner. Otherwise use an acid anti-oxy conditioner to return the hair to its natural acid state and close the cuticle scales.

Lightening and colouring products

There are many different types of colour that can be used depending on whether the client requires something long-lasting or just a temporary measure.

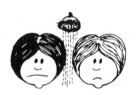

Temporary colours

Temporary colours are very popular because they create an **instant** colour change. They are quick to apply and easy to remove if the client is dissatisfied with the result.

Temporary colours are useful for adding stronger **tones** to natural or artificially coloured light or dark hair, e.g. warm golden, ashen, rich auburn.

Sometimes natural white hair or bleached hair looks too yellow or golden (brassy) and benefits from being neutralised by silver tones.

However, blending in a few grey hairs may be more difficult – remember that grey hair consists of white and naturally coloured hair mixed together. Some colours produce unwanted warm (orange/red) overtones on white hair.

Temporary colours can also be used to darken natural and artificially coloured hair.

The chemistry of temporary colours

The **pigment molecules** of temporary colours are **too large** to enter the hair shaft, so they coat the outside of the hair. This is why they are washed away so easily.

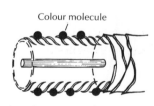

Colour molecule

The chemistry of temporary colours

However, unevenly porous hair (e.g. permed and highlighted ends) will always take a temporary colour unevenly. The cuticle scales are swollen and open in porous hair and the large colour molecules can become trapped and not wash out.

Semi-permanent colours

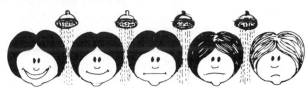

Semi-permanent colours have the advantage of colouring and conditioning hair at the same time. They do not need to be mixed with hydrogen peroxide and so do not leave any regrowth.

They are useful for blending in a small amount of white (grey) hair, but are not strong enough colours to cover a lot of white hair.

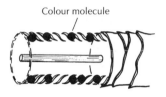

The chemistry of semi-permanent colours

The chemistry of semi-permanent colours
The pigment molecules of semi-permanent colours are **smaller** than those of temporary colours and so are able to penetrate a **little way** into the **cortex** of the hair. They tend to wash out slowly and so last longer than temporary colours.

Unevenly porous hair (e.g. permed, relaxed or bleached hair) will also take a semi-permanent colour **unevenly**. The **cuticle scales are swollen and open** in porous hair and the smaller molecules can penetrate deeper into the cortex in the porous part of the hair, although they rinse off normally from the non-porous parts – producing patchy results.

Quasi-permanent colours

Some of the newer semi-permanents now last up to 15 shampoos because they contain a stronger ingredient called **para**. For these, the client must have a skin test. These colours are different because they are always mixed with a low strength of hydrogen peroxide and are known as **quasi-**, or sometimes **oxy-permanents**. They give a better coverage of white hair and an excellent shine, but can leave a slight regrowth.

Permanent colours

There are three main types of permanent hair colour.

Natural vegetable dyes
The most common of these is **henna**, which gives copper or red tones to the hair. It works by coating the hair shaft and sticking to the outside cuticle layer.

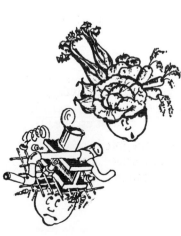

Metallic dyes
These are sold in shops as hair **colour restorers** (e.g. Grecian 2000). **Never perm, tint or bleach over hair coloured using metallic dyes** as it can

break off as a result of the hydrogen peroxide in tint, bleach or neutralisers reacting with the metal salts deposited within the hair by the metallic dye.

Synthetic dyes

Permanent tints are **para** dyes and are known as **oxidation dyes** because they are always mixed with hydrogen peroxide.

The widest possible choice of colours is available with permanent tints. They can be used to darken or lighten (up to four shades lighter), and have a whole range of subtle and vibrant tones.

To do

- Re-read the section in Chapter 1 on incompatibility tests (page 26).

Forms of tint available

Creams (tube)
These are mixed to a creamy consistency and are particularly good for covering coarse, resistant hair.

Oil-based tints (bottle)
These liquids mix to a gel-like thickness and give a more natural finished look.

Oil/cream emulsion (tube/bottle)
These have the benefits of both creams and gel tints and are easy to work with.

The chemistry of permanent tints

Tints are alkaline so will swell the hair and **open up the cuticle scales**, allowing the colour to enter the **cortex**.

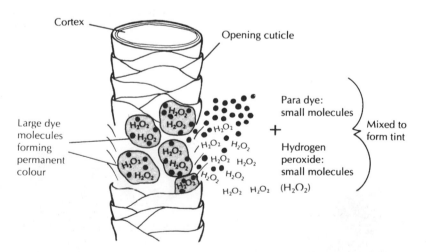

The chemistry of permanent colours

All tints are made of small molecules of **para dye** mixed with **hydrogen peroxide**. These small molecules of tint **link** with the hydrogen peroxide inside the hair shaft to form larger molecules which cannot escape. This is called an **oxidation reaction**.

Once the colour has developed it remains permanently inside the hair shaft, and an **acid anti-oxy rinse** is applied after shampooing to close down the cuticle scales.

| To do |

■ Contact various manufacturers' representatives and technicians to discuss the range of colouring products they offer.

Conventional colouring and bleaching techniques

Remember

Always protect your skin by wearing gloves when applying bleach or colour.

Remember

It is important to consider the image of the client when colouring hair. You need to ensure that the new colour will complement and enhance the personality and appearance of the client and also suit her/his lifestyle.

The following techniques can be carried out on a daily basis in the salon and used to create commercial results.

Woven highlights and lowlights

These are done with foil, 'Easi-Meche' or colour wraps – or, if lowlighting only, a spatula (made by Wella) can be used. Preparing woven highlights is a highly skilled technique.

Prepare the hair by sectioning in the 'nine-section' method so that you can work methodically, step by step. Take sub-sections of hair of a similar size to those used for perming, and weave out the hair with a pin-tail comb. Place the woven strands onto the correct length of foil or Easi-Meche, apply bleach, then re-seal the packets. Always start from the nape and work upwards.

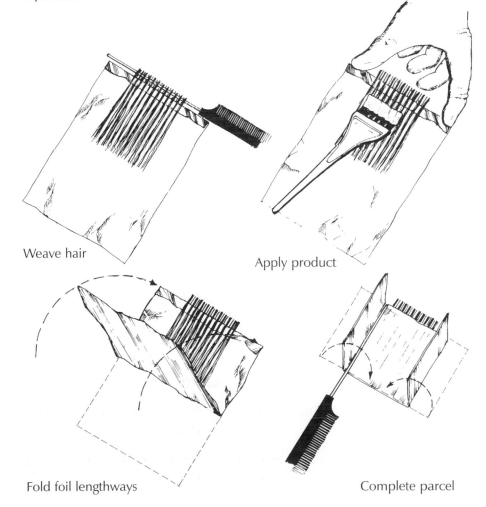

Weave hair

Apply product

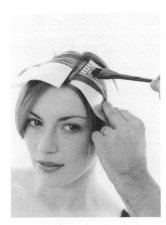

Using colour wraps

Fold foil lengthways

Complete parcel

75

When weaving out the strands of hair, always check that the strand directly below is woven, or the client will end up with stripes. As this is a lengthy process, some of the highlights may develop to the required degree of lightness before completion, so check the development continually. If some highlights are ready, then stop the development on those strands only with cotton wool and warm water.

You might have to re-mix some fresh bleach if it takes you a long time (i.e. over 45 minutes) to complete the head, as the bleach mixture loses its strength after a time.

The advantage of woven highlights is that they are more comfortable for the client. They also allow you to see exactly where the highlights are being placed, and to mix tint and bleach highlights. The product can also be applied closer to the root area than with the cap method.

To do

- Practise woven highlights on models who can spare the time, using thick conditioning cream instead of bleach.

Lowlights

Lowlights are colours which are darker or have more tone than the client's natural base shade (e.g. golden, warm, red or silver). These are applied in the same way as woven highlights. Often two or three colours are used together for woven highlights to give many varied and natural effects. For instance, gold, copper, and light red colours woven alternately on to a dark blonde base can look particularly good.

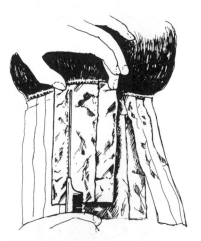
Bleach highlights with foil

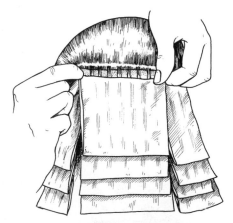
Tint lowlights with adhesive strips

Whole-head tint application

For a whole-head application the tint is always applied to the **mid-lengths and ends**, then to the roots of the hair, unless the hair is very short. This is because heat from the client's scalp makes the tint take more quickly on the roots, which speeds up the processing time. Apply tint to mid-lengths and ends of hair and leave to develop for **half the development time**. Mix up fresh tint and apply to the **root area**, develop for a further 30 minutes

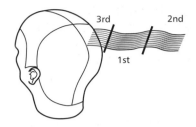

and then remove. This method is used when **lightening** or using **red/copper shades**. When tinting hair **darker**, the colour can be applied from roots to ends in one application.

Developing and timing the tint

- Make sure that the hair is sufficiently **loosened** to allow the circulation of air.
- Check the manufacturer's instructions to see **how long** it should be left before checking (the average time is 30 minutes), and whether you should use **heat** (from an accelerator), which will halve the development time.
- Check the colour development by taking a **strand test**. Remove some of the colour from the roots and the ends and compare the two colours. If they are of the required shade, then remove the colour.

Removing the tint

Take the client to the wash-basin and add a small amount of water to loosen the colour whilst massaging the head. Rinse off the tint thoroughly with tepid water until the water runs clear. Using a cream or an **acid-balanced shampoo**, massage gently, then rinse. Apply a second shampoo if necessary.

Use an acid **anti-oxy conditioning rinse** to prevent the tint from oxidising any further and to close the cuticle scales. Complete the record card.

Alternative techniques

These can be used to enhance fashion styles for more adventurous clients and adapted to produce a variety of results.

Random highlights

For a step-by-step explanation of the technique used to create this effect see colour plate 6.

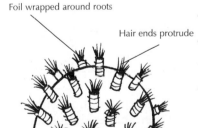
Foil wrapped around roots
Hair ends protrude

Tipping

This creates blond/lighter effects on the tips of the hair to emphasise the shape of the haircut.

This technique can be combined with full-head colouring on short hair. After applying tint, prepare hair as above and process, while tint is still on hair.

When lift is achieved, rinse out bleach and emulsify the tint through to the ends of the hair for 5–10 minutes. This will give the hair the same tone but lighter depth than the roots.

Method
Take triangular sections of hair, pull into an **upright position** and wrap foil around **mid-lengths and roots** to make the hair stand on end. When all areas to be coloured are prepared in the same way, apply bleach or lightening tint to the hair ends and process until desired degree of lift is achieved.

Remember

Always check the manufacturer's instructions relating to product application before starting.

Scrunch colouring

This technique is best suited to curly styles.

Method
- Dry the hair in the desired style
- Mix colouring/lightening product
- Put on plastic/rubber gloves and paint colour onto **palms and fingers**
- 'Scrunch' the colour onto the hair
- Repeat the process until all areas are coated with colour. Leave to process until the desired shade is achieved, then remove the colour

Block colouring

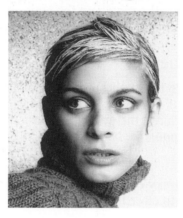

This involves colouring or bleaching sections of hair to create a contrast. The size of the sections taken will depend on the hairstyle and desired result. **Thin sections** will give a **subtle** effect, **thicker** sections will give a **bolder**, **more dramatic** result. See colour plate 7.

Method
- Once you have decided on the areas of hair to be coloured, section the hair as appropriate, ensuring that any hair **not to be coloured** is **clipped out of the way**.
- If colouring a small amount of hair, place a strip of foil under the section, apply colour or bleach and fold foil as for **foil highlighting**, to cover the hair. Leave to process and remove as per manufacturers' instructions.
- If colouring a large block of hair, after sectioning, apply colouring product to the whole section as if colouring a full head.

Graduated/tier colouring

This technique is carried out using three different colours, starting with a **darker** colour in the **nape area** and grading to **lighter shades** throughout the **mid** and **top areas** of the head. The technique is best suited to **graduated hairstyles** which are cut shorter into the nape.

Method
Divide the head into three separate areas using zigzag sections. Apply the darkest colour to the nape area. Once this is completed apply the mid-shade to the central section. Finally, apply the lightest shade to the top area and process as normal.

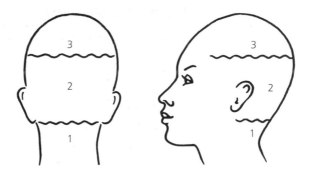

Tier colouring and sectioning

Back to back slices

This technique can create **dramatic results** on **medium to long layered styles** and is best used on the **top section** of the hair. It can be carried out using a variety of colours depending on client requirements.

Method

Take a section through the top of the head **no longer than the width of a foil strip**. Starting on the front hairline weave and wrap the section as for foil highlights. For the next section, take a fine slice of hair, place foil underneath and paint on colour, then place another piece of foil directly on top of the colour. Take the next slice of hair and lay it onto foil, apply colour and place foil on top (like a sandwich with the hair as the filling) alternate colours should be used for best results. Continue in this manner throughout the top section of the hair.

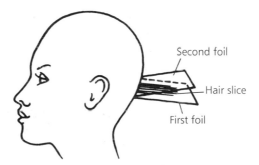

Back to back slices

Tip: To prevent foil slipping slide your tail comb along the foil to make it stick to the hair beneath.

To do

- Think of ways you could enhance the hairstyles of your existing clientele through the use of conventional or fashion colouring techniques.
- Make a list of the tools and equipment you could use to carry out the techniques listed above.

Colour correction

There are many categories of colour correction, from simple examples such as colour fade, seepage of lightening products when highlighting or hair which has become highly lightened by the sun, to the more complex types

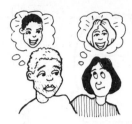 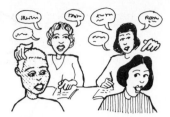 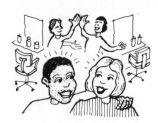

of colour correction and colour removal techniques. Colour removal can be used for a variety of reasons, from removing tone or green discoloration from the hair to removing a build-up of dark colour. Colour removal can be used to remove semi-permanent, quasi- and permanent colours from hair. Reasons for carrying out colour removal include unsuccessful results when hair is tinted, the client wanting to change his or her hair colour, or even to recolour hair after a competition.

In some cases total colour removal is necessary, in others the hair may need to be lightened by only a few shades to remove depth or the intensity of red/copper tones.

Before attempting any type of colour correction, consider the following points:

- **Don't promise anything** to the client – analyse the hair and give realistic advice as to what can be achieved.
- Whatever you decide to do, keep it simple and commercial – it may be easier to restyle the hair than to carry out expensive treatments that may need to be repeated frequently.
- If you do decide to go ahead with major colour removal or correction work prepare your client – advise of the **likely duration** and **costs** of the service(s) being carried out, and whether they will need repeat appointments.
- **Let the client know of any drastic changes to expect** – e.g. going from blonde to red before arriving at the target shade – this will help prevent shocks later.
- Finally, make sure that you get a **level of commitment** from the client – you need to know that, if a series of expensive treatments is required, the client will be committed to seeing them through.

During consultation gain as much information about the hair as possible. If in doubt carry out a test cutting and assess results. Once you begin your service talk the client through what you are doing, reassess the hair at each stage and keep checking stages after application – your options could change as the work progresses.

Once colour correction work is complete always recommend aftercare products and services in order to maintain the finished result.

Types of colour removal product

Colour reducers
Sometimes called **colour strippers**, these remove **artificial colour pigment** only, by breaking down the large colour molecules into smaller ones which are easily washed from the hair.

Remember

Plan your time effectively. Look at salon time available and, where possible, try to book the appointment on a different day to the consultation as this will allow you to allocate enough time to do the job and give you time to prepare. It also gives the client a chance to prepare for the changes that will take place.

To do
■ Read manufacturers' instructions on how to use colour reducers.

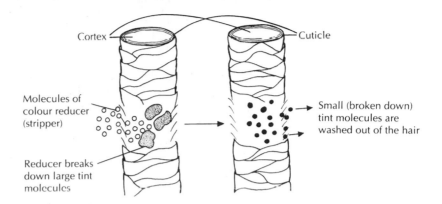

The chemistry of colour strippers

Bleach or oxidation-type products
These are bleaching agents that work in the same way as most bleaches, and remove natural colour pigment as well as artificial colour pigment.

Contra-indications to colour removal

The following circumstances would prevent colour removal taking place:

- Presence of **contagious** or **infectious** conditions of the hair and scalp.
- Hair that has **poor elasticity** or is **highly porous**.
- **Incompatible chemicals** have been used on the hair, for example, products containing **metallic salts**.
- A client who shows a **positive reaction** to a **skin test**.
- A **poor colour result** on a **strand test**.
- A client with a very **sensitive scalp**.
- A **build-up of dark products** on the hair, which would be difficult to remove.

Before starting:

- Carry out a thorough **client consultation**, including colour analysis, and ensure that the client is happy with the chosen colour.
- Make sure that the hair is in **good condition** before starting.
- Always carry out **appropriate tests** – porosity, elasticity, skin, incompatibility and strand tests – and ensure results are **satisfactory** before colour removal.
- Make sure that both you and the client are **well protected**.

During the process:

- Do not allow any **metallic objects** to come in contact with the products being used.
- Always work **methodically** and **quickly**.
- **Never** allow the product to come into **contact with any hair not being**

81

treated. When de-colouring specific areas, **block off any hair not to be treated**.

- **Check** application **thoroughly**.
- **Avoid** the use of a **steamer** for processing as this could cause the product to become diluted or run onto hair not being treated.
- Treat the hair and scalp **gently** when removing product.
- Pay attention to Health and Safety and **COSHH regulations** regarding yourself and your client at all times.
- Always give **after-care advice**. Remember, the client's hair is now highly processed and must be treated with care.

Lightening artificial colour

To remove unwanted tone
This method will not lighten hair colour but removes unwanted tone – for example, ash tones, chlorine green or build up of temporary colour.

Method
Mix one scoop of powder bleach with 60 ml warm water. Pre-shampoo and towel dry the hair, then apply the mixture to the hair using a sponge. Develop visually by watching until unwanted tone is removed. Once the desired amount of colour has been removed shampoo and condition hair.

To remove depth and tone
A cleansing shampoo, or bleach bath, can be used to remove depth and tone and is particularly good for removing red tones.

Method
Mix one scoop powder bleach with 60 ml warm water, 15 ml shampoo and 30 ml 6% hydrogen peroxide. Pre-shampoo and towel dry the hair then apply the mixture to the hair using a sponge (remember this mixture is quite runny) on the areas needing colour removal. Visually develop as before – look for the shade of lift required. If the desired lift is not achieved after 30 minutes, remove and re-apply (you can reduce the amount of water to 30/40 ml for the second application). Rinse off and assess result – if happy, shampoo and condition hair as normal.

To remove maximum depth and tone
Full-strength bleach can be applied to the hair – but this can be used only if the hair condition is very good and test cuttings show a positive colour result.

Pre-pigmentation

This is a technique used to replace **yellow**, **orange** or **red** pigments into bleached hair before tinting the hair back to its natural base. If this is not done, the resulting colour will be **green** or **ashen**.

When carrying out pre-pigmentation, always refer to the manufacturer's instructions for the most suitable method of application, as this can vary from product to product.

Below are two examples of pre-pigmenting techniques.

> **Remember**
>
> You may need to pre-pigment the hair before re-colouring with target shade.

> **Remember**
>
> When using a bleach-type product, do not apply to root area if regrowth is present – it will bleach the natural colour.

> **Remember**
>
> The pre-pigment colour chosen will depend on how dark or light the target colour is. Light bases will need a yellow tone, medium shades a copper tone and dark shades will need a red tone.

Methods

1 Apply a **yellow, orange or red-toned semi-permanent** to the hair and develop. Blot off excess colour with cotton wool. Apply chosen permanent colour and process as normal.

2 Use a permanent colour with a strong yellow, orange or red tone mixed with water. Apply to dry hair, blot off excess product and apply the chosen target shade.

Pre-softening

This is carried out before tinting very resistant hair to ensure good coverage and a satisfactory end result.

Method

Apply 20 vol. (9%) hydrogen peroxide to the resistant areas, using a tinting brush or cotton wool. Place the client under a pre-heated hood dryer, or accelerator, until the hair is dry, then proceed with the tint application as normal.

Tip: Cream peroxide is easier to use and control than liquid peroxide.

> **Remember**
>
> Always use a base shade one shade lighter than required as porous hair will produce a darker result.

> **Remember**
>
> As when pre-pigmenting, always check the manufacturer's instructions for the best possible method of pre-softening.

Counteracting colour fade

There are many causes of colour fade, these include porosity of hair and the effects of sun and sea. The **method used** to counteract colour fade will depend on the **amount of fade** that has taken place.

Minimum fade

This is when the hair has **lost tone** only. The technique used is often called a 'comb through' and can be carried out in a variety of ways, one example of which is given here.

Method

Apply tint to **root area** as normal. Once this colour has developed sufficiently, dampen the ends of the hair using water and **massage** the tint through **from the roots** to the ends of the hair. As the tint is alkaline and will cause the cuticle, or outer layer, of the hair to swell and open, it is advisable not to comb the hair too much at this stage. A good tip is to **use the back of a wide-toothed comb** to **spread the colour** and **avoid damaging the hair**. Once the tint is evenly distributed, leave to process for 5–10 minutes, carry out a strand test to assess results and then remove the tint as per the manufacturer's instructions.

Medium fade

In this instance the hair has lost **depth of colour** as well as tone.

Method

Mix tint and apply to root area as normal. Immediately you have done this, mix up a colour rinse consisting of 60 ml warm water, 15 ml 9% (20 vol.) hydrogen peroxide and 15–30 ml of tint; the amount of tint used will depend on the shade of colour being used – for strong red or copper shades use more tint in the mixture. This formula can be mixed in a bowl and applied with a tint brush or an applicator flask. Apply product straight through mid-lengths and ends of the hair and leave to develop for 30 minutes. Carry out a strand test after developing to assess results then remove product, shampoo and condition the hair as usual.

Maximum fade

For extreme loss of depth and tone an **anti-fade colour bath** is required. This process involves two stages.

Stage 1

As for previous processes, apply tint to root area. Immediately mix 45 ml of warm water with 15 ml of tint and apply to the mid-lengths and ends of the hair; again, if using a strong red shade the mixture can be altered to 30 ml tint and 30 ml warm water. Develop for 30 minutes.

Stage 2

Stabilise the colour by using a mixture of 40 ml warm water and 10 ml 9% hydrogen peroxide to expand the colour molecules, thus making the colour permanent. Pour the mixture through mid-lengths and ends of the hair and work it in with the fingers. Leave for 5 minutes to develop, rinse to remove and shampoo and condition the hair as normal.

Remember
If the client has an ash-toned colour substitute this with a natural shade for the colour bath as the hair can be left with a grey/green cast.

To do
■ Check the manufacturers' instructions of the tinting products you use for their guidelines on dealing with colour fade.

HEALTH MATTERS
When preparing tints, bleaches or colour reducers, always mix in a well-ventilated area.

Colouring and bleaching faults and corrections

Fault	causes	correction
Hair damage/breakage.	Applying bleach (overlapping) onto previously bleached hair. Incorrect proportions of mixture or too many boosters/activators used. Too high a concentration of hydrogen peroxide used. Over-developing the bleach, leaving it on too long (often due to not taking a strand test). Processing with too much heat.	Re-condition the hair and apply restructurants.
Skin/scalp damage.	Not using barrier cream around the hairline. Use of too strong a bleach mixture. Over-developing the bleach: leaving it on too long. Cuts and abrasions on the scalp before bleaching.	If just a little sore, then apply a soothing moisturising cream. If very inflamed, seek medical attention.

Colouring and bleaching faults and corrections (cont.)

Fault	Causes	Correction
Hair not light enough.	Client's base colour too dark for the strength of bleach mixture used. Bleach mixture too weak: peroxide strength too low. Insufficient development time: bleach not left on long enough.	Test hair elasticity and porosity: if satisfactory then re-bleach. Apply a silver, ash or matt toner (for yellow, orange or red hair tones).
Hair over-lightened.	Use of too strong a bleach mixture. Over-developing the bleach: leaving it on too long.	Re-condition the hair, apply restructurants. Re-colour under supervision.
Uneven bleaching result.	Uneven application. Overlapping. No allowance made for body heat on a whole-head application. Bleach mixed badly, lumps left in the mixture. Sections too large. Application too slow.	Spot-bleach darker areas and re-bleach if under-processed.
Hair accepts pre-pigment colour but not target shade.	Hair may be overprocessed.	Re-colour using half base shade + half target shade
Colour result does not match target shade.	Colour under-processed (not timed accurately). Wrong strength of peroxide used. Wrong colour chosen. Client's natural base too dark for colour chosen.	Re-tint hair.
Patches of colour at root area after highlighting.	Colour has seeped during bleaching.	Spot-colour using tint to match natural base.
Result too yellow after bleaching.	Bleach underprocessed/too weak peroxide strength used.	Re-apply bleach and process until desired result is achieved.
Uneven result when tinting.	Uneven application. Sections too wide. Colour mixed incorrectly.	Spot-colour areas that have been missed.
Skin staining.	Poor application of product. Barrier cream not used before applying colour.	Use stain-removal product.

To do

- List the limits of your authority when dealing with problems when colouring and who you would refer a problem to if you could not deal with it yourself.

Test your knowledge

1 Why is it important to carry out hair and skin tests **before** and **during** colouring processes?

2 What **personal protective equipment** should be used when colouring, and why?

3 How should you **dispose** of any unused colouring products?

4 Why is it important to **notify stock shortages**?

5 List three methods of **sterilising** that can be used.

6 Why is it important to **position equipment** for ease of use?

7 Why should you consider the **image of the client** when colouring hair?

8 Why is it important to consider the **image of the salon** when carrying out colour work?

9 When would you use **pre-pigmentation**?

10 Why would you **pre-soften** hair?

11 Give reasons for carrying out a **colour removal or correction**.

12 List the **common colouring faults** and how to correct them.

13 List and describe the range of **colouring and lightening products** available for use.

14 Why must you be aware of the **limits of your own authority** when dealing with problems during colouring?

5 Salon profitability

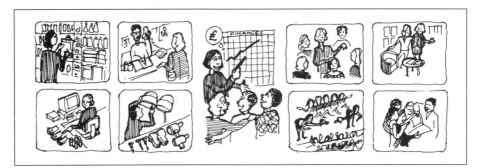

Salon profitability

The financial success of a salon is the responsibility of all staff, from the receptionist and trainee/apprentice to senior management. Contrary to popular belief, salon owners do not use salon takings just to pay staff wages and commission and keep the rest for themselves! The salon takings also go towards the fixed costs of the salon. A salon must have sufficient income to cover salon expenses such as:

- Rent
- Council Tax
- Lighting and heating
- Electricity
- VAT
- National Insurance contributions
- Telephone
- Stationery
- Insurances
- Advertising
- Bank charges
- Stock
- Accountancy
- Sundries, e.g. laundry costs, refreshments
- Cleaning
- Repairs

The biggest percentage of salon income is taken up by salon wages, rent, Council Tax and utilities – water and electricity – with other items on the list taking a smaller percentage.

To do

- Using the headings above, try to work out what percentage of salon income would be taken by each of the items listed.

The financial status and prosperity of any salon will be affected by many factors. Seasonal variations will affect client numbers and profits, but the salon overheads will remain the same even when takings are down. This chapter will concentrate on ways of ensuring effective use of salon resources and maintaining productivity levels.

Resources

There are many different types of resources used in a salon, including human resources (both staff and clients), stock (for retail and professional use), tools and equipment, utilities, fixtures and fittings, information systems, time, space and, most importantly, **money**. All these resources must be used to their fullest potential **at all times by all salon staff**.

To do

- Give examples of resources which may come under each of the categories listed above.
- Within your salon structure, to whom would you report any recommendations for improvements in the use of resources?

Dealing with resources

When dealing with resources, it is important to remember the following:

- Resources should be used for **approved purposes only** – for example, the salon telephone should be used for business calls only and not for staff to ring friends.
- Resources must be used to **best effect**.
- **Wastage** of products and resources, for example, hot water supply, **must be minimal**.
- The use of resources should comply with **organisational** and **legal requirements**. All stock and equipment must be stored, used, handled and disposed of (where applicable) according to manufacturers' instructions, salon and health and safety policies.
- The **misuse of salon resources** could result in wastage, financial loss to the business, damage to tools and equipment, and inconvenience to both clients and staff.

Effective use of resources

To ensure effective use of resources, staff training is essential.

Effective training will ensure that all staff know **how** and **when** to use resources **correctly**, that they comply with **Health and Safety regulations** relating to use of resources and can also instruct others in the use of resources – for example, by teaching junior members of staff how to use products and equipment, or by giving clients after-care advice on products to use in the home.

Finding information

Information on use of resources can be obtained from various sources:

- Product manufacturers
- Training courses and seminars
- Equipment manufacturers
- Instruction leaflets/manuals
- Salon managers/trainers
- Colleges of further education

Staff training

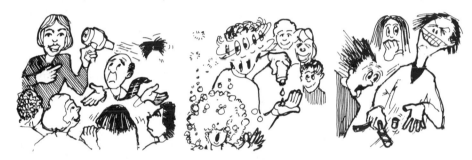

Staff training should take place on a **regular basis**, with health and safety training being updated frequently. Most salons will have staff who have specific responsibilities for training other members of staff, and this training should involve not just teaching new hairdressing skills and techniques, but also **how to deal with clients** and **use new products or equipment**.

To do

- Make up a chart showing who is responsible for the various types of staff training sessions which take place in your salon, under the following headings:
  - Health and safety
  - Equipment/product knowledge
  - Practical skills
  - Client care

Legislation relating to resources

There is a large volume of **legislation** relating to the use of resources in hairdressing, and it is important that all members of salon staff are aware of current laws and that **Health and Safety requirements** are enforced at all times (see Chapter 6, pages 99–122). In addition to Health and Safety legislation, most organisations have their own rules and regulations relating to the use of resources.

Staffing structure

Each salon should have a **staffing structure**, usually consisting of salon owner or manager, senior and junior stylists, trainees or apprentices and, in some cases, a receptionist. Each member of staff should have specific responsibilities within the organisation.

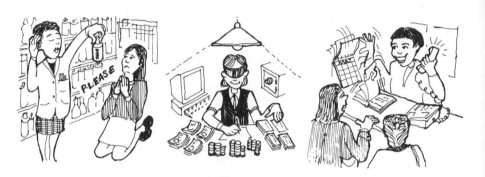

The responsibilities of each member of staff relating to the use of resources should be **clearly outlined** in their job description. It is also a good idea to display a chart in the staff room showing who is responsible for specific resources. Although the salon owner or manager will usually have overall responsibility, each individual member of staff will need a degree of responsibility in order to carry out their daily salon duties. For example, who is responsible for allocating clients (the most important resource of all) to salon staff? Is this done by the receptionist, or are all staff allowed to take bookings?

Problems which may arise

It is important that salons have proper procedures for dealing with any problems which may arise relating to the use of resources, and that all staff are aware of the limits of their authority. They should also know who to refer a problem to if they cannot deal with it themselves.

Listed below are some problems and suggested precautions.

Problem	Preventive measure
Shortage of change in till.	Ensure adequate change in float at beginning of day. Keep change in safe in case of emergencies.
Client in dispute over payment.	Ensure client is informed of salon charges during consultation, before service being carried out.
Running out of stock.	Ensure stocktaking is carried out on a regular basis – weekly/fortnightly.
Discrepancies in amount of takings.	Keep accurate records of money taken in till, together with client bills to cross-check.
Too much shampoo being used.	Ensure staff are aware of correct quantities of shampoo to use.
Hot water being wasted at basins.	Ensure all staff know to turn water off between shampoos.

To do

■ Think of some other problems which could arise relating to resources, and how you could prevent/resolve them.

Productivity in the salon

Poor quality of service, ineffective use of salon resources and failure to make use of opportunities which arise in the salon to offer clients additional services will all result in a **decrease in productivity** within the salon.

Many salons pay staff a commission on their takings and set targets or goals in the form of services to clients or retail sales which the stylist must achieve on a weekly or monthly basis in order to earn their commission.

Setting targets

When setting targets for productivity, it is better to set **small goals** which can be achieved by staff and gradually increased than to set unrealistic targets. For example, junior staff could be set retail targets.

Remember to set the targets in **negotiation with staff** rather than just telling them what you expect – they should be acceptable to both parties. Team goals or targets can be set alongside individual targets, with all salon staff benefiting from their achievement.

Both staff and the salon manager/owner should be responsible for tracking targets throughout the agreed time span, and **time should be set aside** for **regular review meetings**. These review meetings are ideal opportunities for individuals to recognise personal strengths and weaknesses within their existing skills and knowledge and enable them to identify any training needs in order to overcome these weaknesses. Ways of identifying one's own strengths and weaknesses include assessing performance against the targets and goals that have been set – are you doing better in some areas than others? Why might this be? Do you need additional training in order to achieve the targets that have been set? If yes, how can you go about getting the training you need? Other ways of helping to focus on strengths and weaknesses include chats and discussions with colleagues and clients. Chapter 14 gives information on setting targets, identifying strengths and weaknesses and individual and staff training needs.

Failure to achieve the agreed targets will affect any commission paid and should be discussed on a one-to-one basis with the individual concerned to find out the reasons for failure. An action plan can then be devised and new targets set.

Repeated failure to achieve targets could result in some form of disciplinary action.

To do

■ Think of some examples of targets that could be set for salon juniors and stylists in your salon.

Time and motion study

A good way of analysing the productivity levels of staff in the salon is to carry out a **time and motion study**.

This involves observing members of staff over a specific period of time, keeping a detailed record of how many times they carry out each type of practical task or service, and how long each service takes.

Example Time and Motion Study*

Week beginning:

	SERVICES				
	Cut and blow dry	Blow dry/set	Perm	Colour	Relaxer
Time allocated*:					
Day/date					
Totals for week:					
Time spent (hours)					

*average time for basic perm/relaxing/colouring techniques – not including processing or drying time
Number of hours worked:

* A full-size photocopiable version of this form appears on page 228.

To do

■ Devise some time sheets to give to staff and carry out a time and motion study in your salon.

The time span for this activity should be **no less than six weeks** and **no more than three months**. Once all the information has been gathered, you can calculate the average productive time, the percentage of perm, colour and styling work being carried out, the average length of time per service, and the average productive time, per staff member. This will enable you to target quiet times and arrange any special offers and promotions around them.

Increasing productivity

Remember

Good communication skills are essential. Always be polite, tactful, factual and honest, whether dealing with staff or clients. This will ensure accurate information is given and a professional salon image is promoted at all times.

There are many potential opportunities to enhance productivity levels within the salon. These include:

● Staff training
● Promotional events
● Advertising

Staff training

All staff should undertake regular training in both **technical skills** and **product awareness** to enable the salon to offer a **complete range of high-quality services**. The more technical services and after-care advice stylists can offer, the more income they will generate. Training junior staff to carry out simple tasks such as conditioning treatments will also help to increase salon income.

Promotional events

Special offers and promotions should not be restricted to the existing clientele but should be aimed at as **wide a cross-section of the public as possible**. Try giving existing clients a discount on salon services when they bring a friend to the salon. In order to be successful, promotional activities or events must be organised in advance. Chapter 10, pages 164–170, deals with planning and organising promotional events.

Advertising

Using advertisements in local papers and in-house promotional materials will help to promote **specific services**, **staff** or **products** and **special offers**. When clients respond to a promotional advertisement, this gives the stylist the opportunity to tell them of other services on offer in the salon that might benefit them.

To do

■ Re-read the section in Chapter 14 which deals with effective communication within the salon.

Confidentiality of information

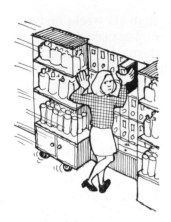

A salon will have many types of information relating to clients and staff, which need to be recorded and updated regularly. The two main ways of recording this information are **manually** through methods such as appointment books, record cards, receipt pads, salon account records, etc., and to use **computerised systems.** Computer packages are available to store client information, staff wage information – pay structures, rates of commission, details of services staff have carried out, stock control – stock levels and order dates, etc. Whichever forms of recording and storing information are used by a salon, it is important that all information kept remains confidential.

To do

- Find out your salon's rules on confidentiality and what could happen if you break them.

Test your knowledge

1 List the **types of resources** available in a salon.
2 What could happen if **salon resources** are **misused**?
3 How can you ensure **correct and effective** use of salon resources?
4 Give examples of how **productivity levels** can be enhanced.
5 What **factors** could affect productivity levels?
6 What could happen if set targets are **not achieved**?
7 Why is **good communication** important?
8 Why should information kept by a salon remain **confidential?**

6 Health, safety and security

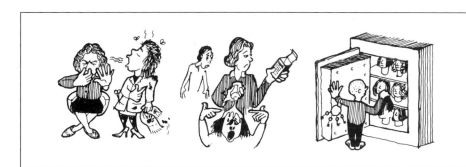

Working practices

Hairdressers must always work:

- **Cleanly**. Both your client's health and your own health are at risk. Tools and equipment must be clean and properly sterilised. There are many diseases that you and your client could catch from dirty equipment – such as headlice, impetigo and ringworm.
- **Safely**. Careless work could lead to hair loss, hair breakage, damage to the client's skin or eyes, or ruined clothes.

Did you know that legally you (the employee) must take care of not only your own health and safety, but also that of anyone else who may be affected by your work?

This means that both you and your staff should:

- Know where the emergency exits are in case of fire, flood, bomb alert or gas leaks
- Know how to telephone for the emergency services (e.g. the fire brigade or ambulance service)
- Know which chemicals used in the salon are dangerous and how to use them safely
- Know how to use electrical equipment safely
- Have some knowledge of emergency first aid
- Work with an awareness of **security procedures**

This applies to:

- Staff and clients, and their possessions
- The salon premises, fixtures and fittings

- Stock, both for salon and retail use
- Suspicious persons and packages

Salon hygiene

In order to prevent the spread of infection:

- Each hairdresser should have at least **two sets of tools**, one in use and the other being sterilised or disinfected ready for the next client.
- **Clean towels and gowns** should be given to each client. Towels should be **washed** and dried after use (not just dried).
- **Hair should be swept up** after every haircut and placed in a covered container.
- All **work surfaces** must be **regularly cleaned** with hot water and detergent. Surfaces should be made of materials that are free of cracks and are easy to keep clean.
- Clients with any **infectious conditions** (e.g. headlice, ringworm or impetigo) **should not be treated in the salon** but tactfully referred to a doctor. If work begins before the problem is noticed, then the service should be completed as quickly as possible. Contaminated hair (e.g. hair containing nits or headlice) should be swept up immediately and preferably burnt; failing this, it should be placed in a sealed container. Hairdressing equipment and clothing that has been in contact with the client must be **sterilised or disinfected**.
- Care should be taken when using **tools which may cut or pierce the skin** or in areas with open, bleeding or weeping wounds or cuts because of the risk of AIDS and Hepatitis B (see below). **Disposable razor blades** must be safely disposed of by placing in a secure container, such as a wide-mouthed screw-topped bottle or **commercial sharps container**, before being placed in the bin.

AIDS (acquired immunodeficiency syndrome)

This is caused by a virus which attacks the natural defence system of the body, preventing it from fighting disease or infection. It is transmitted by blood or tissue fluid from an infected person entering a break in the skin of a healthy person, and can be fatal.

Hepatitis B

This is a virus which attacks the liver. Hepatitis is a very serious disease which can kill. It is transmitted by infected blood or tissue fluid coming into contact with the body fluids of an uninfected person, usually through a cut. Therefore, combs, brushes, etc., should not be used on broken skin affected with boils or skin rashes (such as impetigo) unless they can be sterilised immediately afterwards. If skin is accidentally cut with scissors, clippers or razors, these must immediately be cleaned and sterilised.

Sterilisation and disinfection

All tools such as brushes, combs and hair rollers must be thoroughly **cleaned** with hot soapy water to remove loose hairs, dust and dirt. Scissors and razors can be cleaned with alcohol. This must be done before sterilisation or disinfection.

Sterilisation

This means the killing of all organisms, whether

> **Remember**
>
> If tools are accidentally dropped on the floor, they must be cleaned, dried and sterilised before being used again.
>
> Broken tools must not be used because they can be a source of infection.

- Fungi, e.g. ringworm
- Bacteria, e.g. impetigo
- Parasites, e.g. headlice

Autoclaves

These are highly recommended, as they are the most efficient way of sterilising metal tools, combs and plastics (check beforehand that tools can withstand the heat). Autoclaves sterilise by the creation of steam heat (121°C) and pressure. They take about 20 minutes to work.

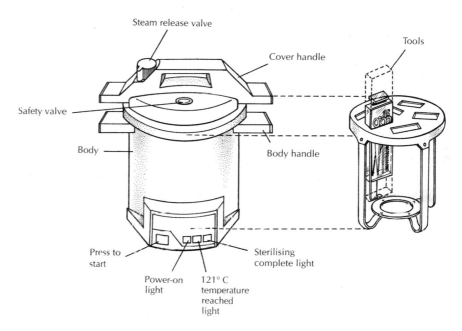

An autoclave

Boiling in water

Towels and gowns should be washed in a hot-wash cycle, where the water should reach 95°C.

Ultraviolet radiation cabinet

These are used in many salons, but all the tools must be perfectly clean before being placed in this cabinet.

During the process, tools must be turned over frequently to expose all surfaces to the ultraviolet rays, which come from a mercury vapour lamp at the top of the cabinet. Each side of the tools should be exposed to the ultraviolet rays for 20–30 minutes.

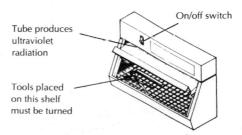

An ultraviolet cabinet

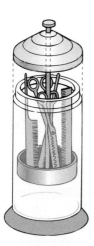

A disinfecting jar

Disinfectants

These chemicals are effective only if used correctly. They quickly become stale or overloaded, and must be used at the **correct concentrations** for the correct length of time.

Personal hygiene and posture

Salon hygiene is extremely important, but **personal hygiene** is equally necessary both for yourself and for your client.

See Chapter 1 regarding personal hygiene (page 5).

Good posture

Good posture not only looks better, allowing clothes to hang properly, but is also more healthy because it allows the bones, muscles, tendons and ligaments to be held in their correct positions, avoiding undue stretching and strain.

Standing correctly

In order to stand correctly, keep the feet hip-width apart, with the weight of the body equally on both legs and the knees slightly bent. Hips and shoulders should be level and the head held up. Common faults are round shoulders, hollow back, and weight held mostly on one foot so that shoulders and hips are tilted.

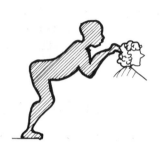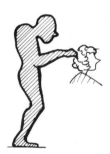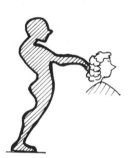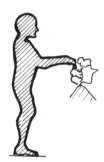

Sitting correctly

In order to sit correctly, the bones should form a right angle at the hip and knee, with the hips and most of the thighs supported by the chair. Common faults are **slouching** (only the base of the spine in contact with the chair so that the back and thighs are not supported) and **crossing the legs**.

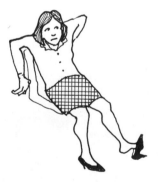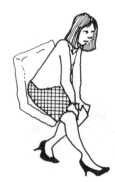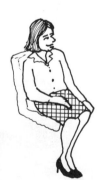

Regular exercise

All muscles need to be worked if they are to remain healthy. If under-used, muscles will begin to weaken and waste away. Regular exercise, such as running, swimming, aerobics and brisk walking will keep the muscles working correctly and help to maintain a good body shape. Exercise will also improve respiration, digestion and blood circulation, as well as relaxing nervous tension.

Safe practices in the salon

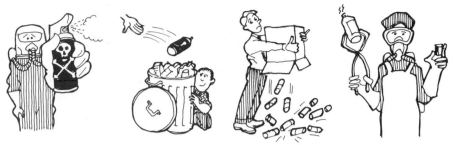

Working safely in the salon is not just a matter of common sense. There are now many **government laws and acts** which are designed to protect **staff**, **clients** and **the environment**.

Here is a brief summary of the main laws and acts that affect hairdressers.

The Health and Safety at Work Act 1974

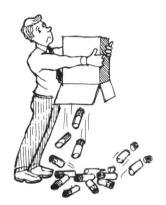

Under the Act, it is the **duty of every employee** at work to take **reasonable care not to endanger the health, safety or welfare of others. Employees must not interfere with or misuse any items** provided in the interests of Health and Safety.

The Manual Handling Operations Regulation 1992

This states that all employees at work have a duty to **minimise the risks from lifting and handling objects**.

The Personal Protective Equipment at Work Regulations 1992

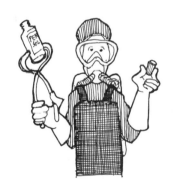

These regulations confirm the requirement for all employers to provide suitable and sufficient **protective clothing**, and for all employees to **use** it when required. In the case of hairdressers, this means wearing protective gloves and tinting aprons when colouring, bleaching, perming and relaxing.

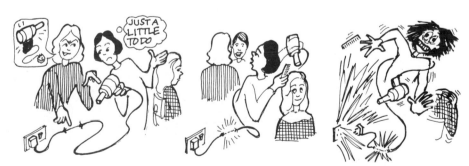

The Provision and Use of Work Equipment Regulations 1992

Under these regulations, employers have a duty to select equipment for use at work which is **properly constructed, suitable for the purpose and kept in good repair**. Employers must also ensure that all who use the equipment have been **adequately trained**.

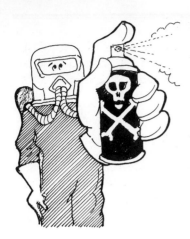

The requirement for competence to use salon tools and equipment is embodied within these hairdressing standards.

The Control of Substances Hazardous to Health Act 1988 (COSHH)

This is enforced by Health and Safety inspectors. It is particularly relevant to the storage and use of hazardous chemicals such as hydrogen peroxide or perm lotions.

It applies not only to you but also to chemicals applied and sold to non-employees, i.e. **clients**.

The Act states that **staff** must be given **information**, **instruction** and **training** on both **hazardous** and **potentially hazardous chemicals** used in the salon.

The HMWA (The Hairdressing Manufacturers' and Wholesalers' Association Ltd) publish an excellent leaflet, *A Guide to Health and Safety in the Salon*, which is available to all salons. There is also a free leaflet, *Five Steps for Completing COSHH Assessments*, which is available from your local Health and Safety Executive (HSE) office.

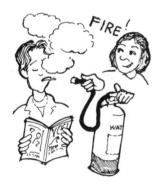

Fire Precautions Act 1971

This is enforced by the local fire authority, usually the fire brigade. It states that all premises must have fire-fighting equipment which is in good working order, suitable for the type of fires which are likely to occur, and readily available. It also states that room contents should be arranged and doors left unlocked to enable a quick exit in case of fire.

The Reporting of Injuries, Diseases and Dangerous Occurrences Regulations 1995 (RIDDOR)

If you, your staff or your clients suffer from a personal injury at work, it must be **reported** in the salon's **Accident Book**. This is in order to inform your employer, and so that serious injuries may be reported to the local Enforcement Office.

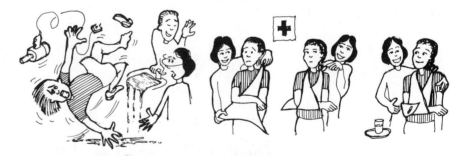

To do
■ It may be that you are responsible for some or all of the areas covered by these Acts. If it is not written in your job description, then ask your salon manager/owner for clarification.

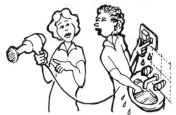

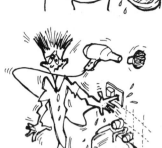

Electricity at Work Regulations 1990

These state that every electrical appliance in a work site must be tested **at least every 12 months** by a qualified electrician. A written record must be kept of these tests, to be shown to the Health and Safety authorities upon inspection.

The Environmental Protection Act 1990

This states that hairdressing salon chemicals (i.e. 'waste') must be disposed of safely – i.e. **poured down the sink** (to dilute and remove them). **Never** put them in the dustbin where they could be found by children.

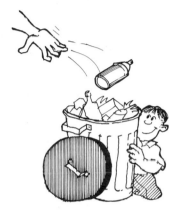

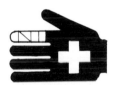

The Health and Safety (First Aid) Regulations 1981

These regulations require every employer to provide **equipment and facilities** appropriate for administering **first aid** to their employees.

Health and Safety at Work Act 1974 (HASAWA)

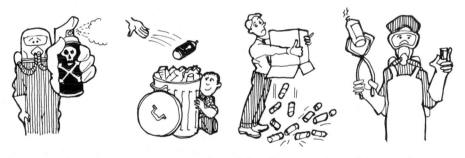

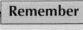

Remember

Local bylaws – salons should register with the local council using form OSR.

This is enforced by Environmental Health Officers and Health and Safety Inspectors. It protects almost everyone involved in working situations. It states the responsibilities of the employer and the employees relating to:

- First aid (emergency aid) arrangements and the reporting of accidents
- General health and safety
- Enforcement of the Act

Penalties and fines

Failure to comply with the Health and Safety At Work Act carries the following penalties and fines:

101

- **Minor** offences, e.g. obstructing an Enforcing Officer: **fines up to £5,000**
- **Serious** offences, e.g. failing to comply with an improvement order from the Enforcing Officer: **fines up to £20,000 and/or six months' imprisonment**
- **Very serious** offences, e.g. resulting in death: **unlimited fines and/or up to two years' imprisonment**

Therefore you must take health and safety seriously.

Health and safety checklist

Does your salon have five or more employees? If so, then you must have a written Health and Safety Policy as shown below.

Health and Safety At Work Act 1974

General Statement of Policy

Our salon's policy is to provide and maintain safe and healthy working conditions, equipment and systems of work for all our employees. We will provide such information, training and supervision as is required for this purpose. We also accept our responsibility for the health and safety of clients and any other people who may be affected by our activities. We will maintain safe access to and egress from our premises at all times.

Name _____

Position _____

Date _____

Review Arrangements

This policy will need to be reviewed at least every six months and amended as required. All members of staff will be involved in the review.

The person responsible for instigating the review is:

Name _____

The Health and Safety Policy must also give details of review arrangements as shown below:

Health and Safety Policy Review Dates*		
	Planned date	*Actual review*
1		
2		
3		
4		

* A full-size photocopiable version of this form appears on page 229.

Also required is a full statement of staff duties and responsibilities with regard to health and safety. An example is shown below.

Health & Safety At Work Act 1974

Statement of staff responsibilities

Overall responsibility for Health and Safety in the salon is that of:

Name _____

Position _____

The person responsible for Health and Safety on a day-to-day basis *(normally you, the supervisor, or manager)* in the salon is:

Name _____

Position _____

In the above person's absence, the following person will be responsible as his/her deputy:

Name _____

Position _____

The person responsible for Health and Safety training is:

Name _____

The person responsible for enforcing salon rules is:

Name _____

The person responsible for First Aid and in particular checking the First Aid box contents and re-stocking as necessary is:

Name _____

The First Aid box is kept: _____

The trained and qualified First Aider is:

Name _____ Type of qualification _____

Certificate number _____ Expiry Date: _____

The person responsible for the Accident Book and for reporting accidents is:

Name _____

The Accident Book is kept: _____

The person responsible for fire safety and in particular checking fire extinguishers, fire exit signs, escape routes and organising fire drills is:

Name _____

The person responsible for providing and replenishing Personal Protective Equipment is:

Name _____

The person responsible for inspecting electrical equipment such as the portable hand tools on a three-monthly basis and adding any new/replacement tools to the checklist is:

Name _____

The person responsible for carrying out, updating and monitoring the COSHH assessments is:

Name _____

The COSHH assessments are kept:

_____

Remember

It is a legal requirement to display the Health and Safety Law poster in your salon.

Day-to-day responsibilities under HASAWA

You will need to know where you can access information on Health and Safety legislation. It may be from:

- Health and safety literature from HSE and the Hairdressing Training Board
- The local library
- Your local council offices
- Reference books

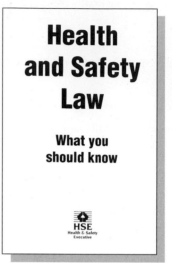

Leaflet published by the Health and Safety Executive

It is also a good idea to produce a chart of **key names and addresses** for quick reference, e.g.:

Health and Safety Policy: Important Contacts*			
Key contact	**Contact name**	**Tel/fax**	**Address**
Environmental Health Officer			
Hospital			
Doctor			
Fire Safety Officer			
Employment Medical Advisory Service			
Local Police Station			

Once you have **collected and itemised** all your information you need to know how to pass this information on to the rest of the staff. You could do this through:

- Staff meetings and verbal discussions
- Training days
- Displaying and/or circulating memos and leaflets (see Salon Rules, page 106)
- Implementing the information in the salon
- By displaying notices such as:

* A full-size photocopiable version of this form appears on page 230.

FIRE DRILL*

IN THE EVENT OF A FIRE

1. TELEPHONE 999 FOR THE FIRE BRIGADE
2. CLOSE ALL DOORS AND WINDOWS
3. LEAVE THE BUILDING BY THE NEAREST EXIT
4. ASSEMBLE OUTSIDE THE SALON

DO NOT

1. STOP TO COLLECT ANY PERSONAL BELONGINGS
2. RE-ENTER THE BUILDING UNTIL THE ALL CLEAR HAS BEEN GIVEN

THE NEAREST EXITS ARE:

THE SALON FRONT DOOR, THE SALON BACK DOOR

---

*IF YOU FIND AN UNATTENDED PARCEL, A SUSPICIOUS OBJECT, OR IF YOU SUSPECT THAT THERE IS LIKELY TO BE AN EXPLOSIVE DEVICE, GAS LEAK ETC. IN OR NEAR YOUR SALON

- DO NOT TOUCH OR MOVE THE PARCEL/OBJECT
- EVACUATE THE SALON
- CALL THE POLICE
- WARN MEMBERS OF THE PUBLIC
- WARN THE OCCUPANTS OF ADJACENT PREMISES

DO NOT RE-ENTER THE AREA UNTIL INSTRUCTED TO DO SO BY THE POLICE

ALWAYS REMEMBER IF IN DOUBT – SHOUT!

You will need to identify your salon's hazards and risks and record them by using this form:

Health and Safety Risk Evaluation*					
	Potential hazard	Degree of risk Low/Med/High (please circle)	Persons at risk	Action need to minimise risk	By when	By whom
1		L M H				
2		L M H				
3		L M H				
4		L M H				
5		L M H				

The management of Health & Safety at Work Regulations 1992

This legislation requires salon owners to maintain and improve health and safety at work, provide proper training and to evaluate risk assessments.

Health and safety training

A lot of **time and money** is spent training someone to become a hairdresser. This would be completely wasted if they end up being unable to work due to **poor health and safety training**.

* Full-size photocopiable versions of these forms appear on pages 232–234.

Salon Rules*

Salon safety and hygiene

Fixtures, fittings, chairs, trolleys and mirrors to be regularly cleaned.

Non-electrical equipment to be kept clean and sterilised at all times.

Electrical equipment to be visually checked for safety, then switched off, unplugged and stored between use.

Floors to be swept clean, free from hair, and spillages immediately mopped up.

Used gowns and towels to be placed in the laundry basket.

Rubbish to be removed immediately and placed in a covered container. Store in sealed rubbish bags while awaiting disposal.

Food and drink must be consumed only in the staff rest room.

Rest room to be kept clean and tidy. Wash up cups, plates and saucers immediately after use.

Staff who smoke must use the smoking area in the rest room.

Stock room to be kept clean and tidy. Stock to be correctly stored and lids and tops replaced immediately after use.

Reception area to be kept clean and tidy.

Fire precautions

Smoking is not allowed in any area of the salon, only outside the back entrance.

Keep all fire exits and egress to them clear at all times.

Do not obstruct fire extinguishers.

Unlock fire exits during working hours.

Security

Keep till drawer locked when not in use.

Keep all stock doors and cupboards locked when not in use.

● Do not bring any valuables to the salon. Keep your purse/money on your person at all times.

Lock all fire exits, close all windows and lock all doors at night.

* A full-size photocopiable version of this form appears on page 231.

Basic health and safety induction should be carried out on the **first day** the employee or trainee starts work and completed **by the end of the first week**.

The induction should cover the following:

- **The salon's Health and Safety policy.** Give the person a copy of the Health and Safety Law leaflet (see page 104) and point out the Key Names and Addresses chart. If you display a Health and Safety law poster, then explain this to them. Also give them a copy of the Salon Rules.

- **Fire precautions.** Explain where the fire extinguishers are kept and how to use them. Point out the fire drill notices and show them where the nearest fire exits are. Tell them who is responsible for fire safety. Note that fire extinguishers colour-coded **blue** (dry powder), **black** (CO_2) and **green** (vaporising liquids) can be used on **electrical fires**. **Red** (water, CO_2, soda acid) and **cream** (foam) must **never be used** on **electrical** fires – water conducts electricity and you will be **electrocuted**.

> **Remember**
>
> This induction must be reviewed every six months.

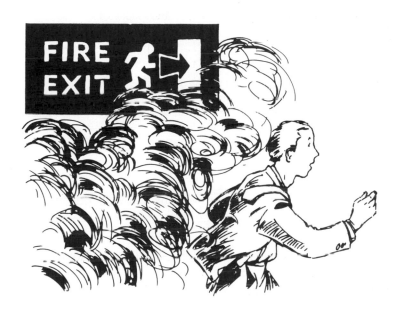

These signs are now mandatory

> **Remember**
>
> Since 1997 European regulations have made all fire extinguishers red with different-coloured labels. **Check the label before using.**

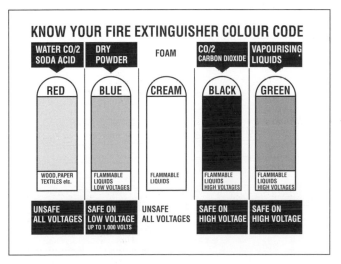

Fire extinguisher codes

- **First aid arrangements.** Tell them who is responsible for first aid in the salon and show them where the first aid box is kept (see page 118).

Explain who is responsible for the reporting of accidents and the Accident Book.

- **COSHH.** Outline the COSHH Act to them and tell them who is responsible for carrying out, updating and monitoring the COSHH assessments.
- **Personal protective equipment.** Show them where the gloves and aprons are kept and when they should be used.
- **Electrical equipment.** Tell them who is responsible for inspecting electrical equipment and what to do if they notice anything that looks dangerous.
- **Contingency precautions.** Show them where the main electricity switch, the water stopcock and the main gas valve are located.

Keep a record of all staff Health and Safety inductions and reviews, e.g.:

			Areas inducted							Health and Safety review dates			
Staff name	Signature	Date	Health & Safety policy and Salon Rules	Fire precautions	First Aid and accidents	COSHH	Personal protective equipment	Electrical equipment	Trainer's signature				

Health and Safety Training Record*

To make sure that the member of staff has understood the induction, ask them to complete the following questionnaire:

Health and Safety Induction Questionnaire*

Name _____   Date _____

1. Who is the main person in charge of Health and Safety in the salon? ....
2. Who is responsible for day-to-day Health and Safety? ....
3. Who does the Health and Safety training? ....
4. Who is in charge of:

	Person responsible	Salon location
a) Salon Rules	....	....
b) First Aid Box	....	....
c) Accident Book	....	....
d) COSHH assessments	....	....
e) Personal Protective Equipment	....	....
f) Fire drills	....	....
g) Notices	....	....
h) Exit signs	....	....

5. Describe the different fire extinguishers:

Colour	Type	Use
....	....	....
....	....	....
....	....	....
....	....	....

* Full-size photocopiable versions of these forms appear on pages 235–237.

The Manual Handling Regulations 1992

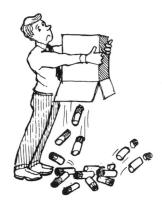

These regulations cover the lifting of loads such as salon stock or video units, as well as lowering, pushing, pulling, carrying and moving them, whether by hand or by using bodily force.

To prevent accidents and injuries when lifting, you should bear in mind the following:

- **The weight of the load.** Try to use a trolley to transport heavy or bulky items into the dispensary and stock rooms. If the package is too heavy for you, either ask another member of staff to help you or unpack the box carefully until it is light enough to be moved.
- **The shape of the load.** Some loads may not be particularly heavy but are bulky and awkward to lift.
- **Distribution of load.** Before attempting to lift, look inside boxes to ensure that the contents are evenly distributed.
- **Your personal limitations.** If you have recently had an illness such as 'flu, you may not have regained your normal strength.
- **Loose items.** Check for loose staples before attempting to lift boxes, and do not put loose items on top of them when lifting.
- **The working environment.** If the area is damp, your hands could be wet and the load might slip.
- **Ease of access.** Will you have to negotiate awkward doorways or stairs?
- **Storage.** Sometimes stock needs to be stored on high shelves. Always use a strong, sturdy step ladder, never a chair or anything unsteady.

Remember

If you send a member of staff to collect equipment or stock from a wholesaler or another salon, make sure that:
- The member of staff has suitable car insurance.
- The member of staff is capable of lifting the equipment or stock without difficulty.

Note: If any member of staff is injured in a road accident whilst on company business, this is now reportable under RIDDOR if they are away from work for more than three days.

Lifting heavy loads

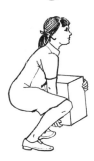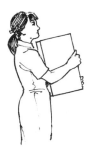

Always lift heavy loads with knees bent and back straight

When lifting, **keep your knees bent** and your **back straight** at all times. If you lift incorrectly you could strain a ligament or a joint in your spine.

- Keep your feet apart, one foot slightly in front of the other to maintain your balance, and face the direction in which the object is to be moved. Never try to lift in a sideways direction.
- Grip the package firmly, keeping it close to your body with your chin tucked well in. Keep the package close to your body, bending at your knees and hips and making sure that your knees are directly above your feet. Allow your strong leg muscles to take the weight, not your back.
- When lowering the object to the ground, be careful to keep your back straight, feet apart and knees and hips bent. Gently does it: remember that **lowering heavy objects can be just as dangerous as lifting them**.

There are five main types of injury which can occur due to manual handling:

- Disc injuries
- Muscular/nerve injuries
- Ligament/tendon injuries
- Hernias
- Fractures, abrasions and cuts

These can all be avoided by observing the above procedure.

The major risk in a salon is from lifting boxes of stock items onto and off shelves. The risk assessment in this case is a very simple one and, although it needs to be carried out, it need not be formally recorded.

Personal Protective Equipment at Work Regulations 1992

The requirements of these regulations will have been met when you comply with your COSHH regulations.

The regulations require employers to provide suitable protective clothing for all employees to use when required. This includes, for example, **wearing protective gloves and tinting aprons when colouring, bleaching, perming and relaxing**.

Staff must be **trained** and **monitored** to ensure that these regulations are properly enforced.

The Provision and Use of Work Equipment Regulations 1992

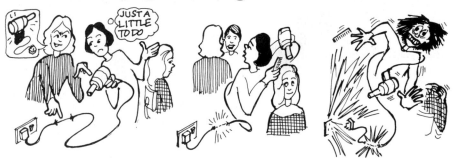

The following requirements apply to all equipment from 1st January 1993:

- **Work equipment must be suitable for the purpose for which it is used.**
- **All equipment must be properly maintained and records kept.**
- **All salon staff must be given adequate health and safety training and written instructions where required.**

To do
Complete the following checklist, ticking if the answer is Yes, taking appropriate action if the answer is No.

- Is all the equipment in my salon regularly checked to make sure that it is in serviceable condition?
- Do I keep maintenance records, particularly for electrical equipment?
- Is second-hand equipment checked by a competent person before use?
- Have all staff been trained in the safe use of all salon equipment?

Electricity at Work Regulations 1990

These regulations cover the installation, maintenance and use of electrical systems and equipment.

The salon's **electrical circuits** and **all electrical equipment** should be tested **at least every 12 months** by a **qualified electrician**. Each electrical hand tool should be listed, numbered and marked with the last test dates.

Schedule of Electrical Items*			
Item	Serial no.	Purchase date	Disposal date
1			
2			
3			
4			

Remember

All tools brought in by members of staff must be numbered, added to the list of items in the Electrical Equipment Register and included in the checks along with any new equipment purchased.

Regular safety precautions should include:

- Removing any **trailing electrical cables** (dry flexes).
- Checking the **temperature controls** before using any equipment, and making sure the **filters** at the back of the hairdriers are **clear and free of dust** to prevent overheating.
- Always **switching off and disconnecting** equipment straight after use.

In addition, a three-monthly visual check on hand tools should be carried out by a member of staff. This should include:

- Looking at equipment to make sure that **flexes and cables** are **not worn or faulty.** Any flexes with worn insulation or any plugs that are **broken or cracked** should be **replaced.**
- Making sure that electrical equipment is **stable.** Check that hairdriers, tongs or hot brushes are safely stored on the work surface and not in places where they are likely to fall off.

Testing Programme for Salon Appliances*							
ELECTRICAL SUPPLIER		TESTING DATES					
Name and address	Tel. No.	Target	Actual	Target	Actual	Target	Actual

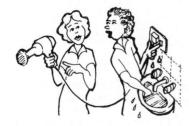

Electric shock

This occurs when a person's body completes an electrical circuit. The size of the shock depends on the size of the electrical current, and can vary from a slight tingling to a cardiac arrest (when the heart stops beating and breathing stops).

* Full-size photocopiable versions of these forms appear on pages 238 and 239.

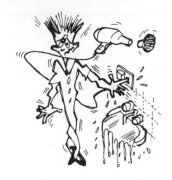

It can happen when a person touches bare wires on flexes or cables, through incorrect wiring or a fault in the plug or appliance, or as a result of touching a switch or plug with wet hands (water acts as a conductor and electricity will flow through the person rather than through the circuit).

Wiring a plug

It is strongly recommended that a residual current device, known as an earth leakage trip, rated at 30mA, be fitted in the circuits to which hand tools are connected.

Make sure you know how to wire a plug correctly:

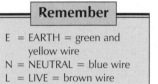

Remember

E = EARTH = green and yellow wire
N = NEUTRAL = blue wire
L = LIVE = brown wire

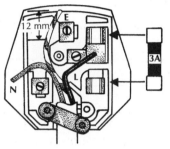

1 Cut away the outer cable, unscrew the cable grip and insert the cable

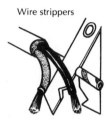

2 Cut away the insulation using wire strippers

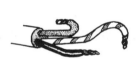

3 Twist the copper strands together

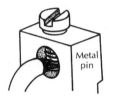

4 Insert each wire into the correct pin

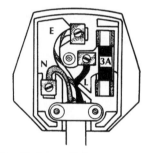

5 Tighten all the screws and the cable grip. Attach the plastic back

The Control of Substances Hazardous to Health Act 1988 (COSHH)

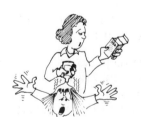

Chemical substances are hazardous by:

- **Inhalation** – breathing in fumes
- **Ingestion** – swallowing them directly or by eating food while chemicals are on the fingers
- **Absorption** – through the skin or via the eyes
- **Contact** – with the skin or eye surface (a chemical of this sort is known as an irritant)
- Being **injected** into the body
- Being introduced into the body via **cuts**, etc.

Basic safety rules for storage of salon chemicals are as follows:

- **Never** use food or drink containers to store any chemical product
- Store products **at or below room temperature** in a **dry atmosphere**, never in direct sunlight, and according to manufacturers' instructions

- Store all **glass** bottles **below eye level**
- Keep products, particularly aerosols, away from naked flames or heat
- Take special care to prevent children gaining access to salon storage areas. **Keep all products out of reach of children**

Mixing chemicals safely

- Follow the **manufacturer's instructions** exactly
- **Dilute** the product according to the manufacturer's recommendations
- **Never mix** products unless this is recommended by the manufacturer
- **Replace all caps and bottletops** immediately to avoid spillage. Make sure unused mixtures and empty containers are disposed of carefully

Using chemicals safely

- Always wear **protective gloves and protective clothing** where indicated (see chart on page 114). Remember that prolonged and frequent use of non-hazardous products such as shampoos may cause dryness and sore skin. To avoid this, wear protective gloves or use **barrier cream** and **moisturiser** as often as possible.
- **Wipe and clean all surfaces where spillages occur.**
  Under the COSHH regulations employers must:
    - **Identify substances in the workplace which are potentially hazardous**
    - **Keep records of manufacturers' data sheets for all chemicals and products and carefully assess any new chemicals and products before use**
- **Assess the risk to health** from exposure to hazardous substances and record the results
- Assess which **members of staff are at risk**
- Look for **alternative, less hazardous substances** and substitute these if possible
- Decide what **precautions** are required, noting that personal protective equipment should be provided free of charge
- Introduce effective measures to **prevent or control exposure to potentially hazardous substances**
- **Inform, instruct and train** all members of staff
- **Review the assessment** on a regular basis.

See the table showing Chemical Hazards and Precautions, page 114.

Controlling the salon environment

This means making sure that the salon does not become **too hot** or **cold** and is **well ventilated** to protect against dangerous fumes.

The Health and Safety at Work Act 1974 states that the working temperature should be 16°C (60.8°F) after the first hour. Precautions should also be taken to avoid salons becoming humid due to hair-drying equipment and steam from hot water supplies, which can also make for difficult working conditions.

To do
Ask staff to find out how to: ■ Operate the salon's heating system through the use of thermostats ■ Ventilate the salon by opening the windows or using the extractor fans.

Ventilation

The COSHH regulations also cover ventilation, especially when mixing chemicals (think about the smell when mixing powder bleach, for instance), so make sure products are mixed in a **well ventilated area**.

Remember also that portable gas or paraffin heaters need proper ventilation to prevent any build-up of irritant gases.

To do

■ Use the COSHH Risk Assessments chart on page 115 to assess your salon's risks.

Chemical hazards and precautions

Chemicals	Health hazard	Precautions
All aerosols, including hairspray	Dangerous if inhaled excessively.	Use in a well ventilated area. Keep well away from lit cigarettes.
	Flammable	Do not tamper with valves: the contents are under pressure and can explode in a fire.
Setting lotions, mousses and gels	Potential irritant	Avoid eye contact.
	Flammable	Keep away from lit cigarettes.
Hydrogen peroxide	Irritant to skin and eyes.	Always wear protective gloves.
		Avoid contacts with eyes and sensitive skin. Replace cap immediately after use.
		Do not allow to mix with other chemicals as it can react and become explosive.
Bleaches	Dangerous if inhaled excessively.	Use in a well-ventilated area.
	Irritant to skin and eyes.	Wear protective gloves.
		Avoid contact with eyes and sensitive skin.
Perm lotions and relaxers	Irritant to skin and eyes.	Wear protective gloves.
		Avoid contact with eyes and sensitive skin.
Perm neutralisers	Irritant to skin and eyes.	Wear protective gloves.
		Avoid contact with eyes and sensitive skin.
Hair colours, tints and semi-permanents	Irritant to skin and eyes.	Wear protective gloves.
	Can cause allergic reactions.	Avoid contact with eyes and sensitive skin.
		Always do a skin test before use.

COSSH Risk Assessment*						
Hazard	What is the risk?	Degree of risk			Who is at risk?	Action to be taken	Date
		High	Med	Low			

Fire Precautions Act 1971

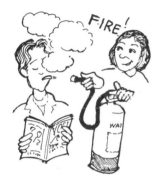

Under this act, a **fire certificate** is required for the premises if:

- **More than 20 people are employed on one floor at any one time**
- **More than 10 people are employed on different floors at any one time**

If the premises are shared with other employers, you must include all people working in the premises when deciding if a fire certificate is required. If your salon is rented or leased, always check with the landlord if a fire certificate is required and if so, whether a certificate has already been issued. Check with the local fire brigade if you have any doubts.

Whether or not a fire certificate is required, **all** premises must be provided with an adequate means of escape and appropriate fire-fighting equipment.

Fire drill notices explaining what to do in case of fire must be **clearly displayed**. All **fire exits** should be **clearly marked** with the appropriate signs.

Staff should not use fire extinguishers unless they have been **fully trained** in their use.

Emergency procedures

You must know how to vacate your building quickly and safely in the case of fire, flood, gas leaks, suspicious packages or a bomb alert, and be able to locate the assembly points outside the salon. You must be aware of where fire-fighting equipment is kept and trained staff know how to use it.

Remember

Fire in the salon may be caused by:
- Incorrect handling of inflammable hairdressing chemicals, such as ethyl acetate (nail polish remover) and hairspray
- Careless cigarette smoking

Fire Equipment Test Record*							
FIRE EQUIPMENT SUPPLIER		TESTING DATES					
Name and address	Tel. No.	Target	Actual	Target	Actual	Target	Actual

* Full-size photocopiable versions of these forms appear on pages 240 and 241.

The Environmental Protection Act 1990

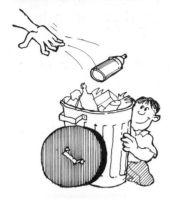

Under this Act, anyone disposing of waste chemicals a matter has a duty of care to ensure all the waste is disposed of **safely**.

For the purposes of the Act, **all the salon's chemicals are considered to be waste**. They must therefore be diluted for disposal – i.e. poured down the sink – thereby **lessening their potential adverse effects on the environment**.

It is important to take care when disposing of surplus or out-of-date stock. Always check with the manufacturers for guidance. If in doubt, ask the manufacturer to dispose of the stock for you.

Remember

Never put chemicals in the dustbin where they could be found by children.

To do

- Ask your product suppliers for advice on the safe disposal of your chemicals and products.
- Check to ensure that all staff know how to dispose of chemicals and products safely.
- Check that all your waste products are kept in a safe place away from children.

The Reporting of Injuries, Diseases and Dangerous Occurrences Regulations 1995 (RIDDOR)

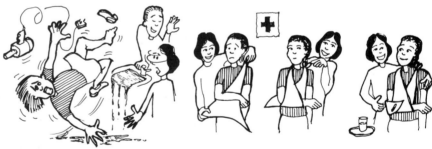

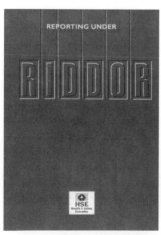

RIDDOR booklet published by the Health and Safety Executive

These regulations require that **if you or your staff suffer personal injury at work** resulting in

1 A **fatality**
2 A **major injury**
3 More than 24 hours in **hospital**
4 **Incapacity** for **more than three calendar days** (excluding the day of injury but including weekends and holidays)

the incident must be **notified in writing** to the local Enforcement Officer.

This is done by completing **form F2508** (copies of which can be obtained from either Dillons Bookshops or direct from HSE books). It should be sent **within seven days of the accident or injury occurring**.

If a client or visiting member of the public should suffer serious injury and be taken to hospital, or die on the premises, **this must also be reported**.

Notifying the Enforcement Officer

For accidents in **categories 1–3** above and **dangerous occurrences** (e.g. a serious fire), the local Enforcement Officer must be **notified quickly** by telephone. This should then be followed up by **form F2508**.

In addition, if **a client or visitor to your premises** suffers **personal injury in categories 1–2** above, this must also be reported to the local Enforcement Officer.

Below is a list of salon services, possible damage and ways of avoiding that damage.

Potential client injury

Client service	Possible injury or damage	Precautions
Styling	Burnt skin or scalp during drying. Damage to clothes from products.	Learn how to work drying equipment. Gown the client, covering all clothes.
Cutting	Cut skin.	Advise client how to sit during cutting.
Colouring and lightening	Allergic skin or scalp reaction. Hair condition deteriorating. Hair breakage. Scalp burns. Damage to clothes from products.	Carry out a skin test. Follow manufacturer's instructions for selection, preparation, development times and removal of products. Gown the client, covering all clothes.
Perming and relaxing	Hair condition deteriorating. Hair breakage. Scalp burns. Damage to clothes from products.	Carry out any necessary pre-treatment tests. Follow manufacturer's instructions for selection, preparation, development times and removal of products. Ensure correct selection of tools and equipment. Use barrier cream. Gown the client, covering all clothes.

Recording accidents

All salon accidents must be reported in the salon's Accident Book. This should be set out as shown on page 118.

It is important to record **all** accidents so that when a review of Health and Safety procedures is carried out (which should include a review of the Accident Book) repetitions can be avoided.

117

Accident Book*					
When did the accident happen? (Give date and time)	**Where did the accident happen?**	**How did the accident happen?** (Give as much detail as possible)	**Name of person(s) involved and nature of injuries**	**Who investigated and reported the accident?** (Give full name and position)	**Was the accident reportable under RIDDOR?**

Remember

The key reason for carrying out an accident investigation is to prevent a re-occurrence – not to decide who is to blame.

To do

■ Remind your staff that all accidents must be recorded in the Accident Book.
■ Check that you have copies of form F2508 available for reporting accidents.
■ Ask staff regularly if they have signs of dermatitis or asthma. If signs of either are detected, then you must take suitable action to minimise the problem, either by providing barrier cream and gloves, or by improving ventilation and seeking medical help.

Occupational dermatitis and **asthma** are also reportable. You may wish to use the following chart for your records:

Asthma/Dermatitis Records*				
Name	**Reported date of symptoms**	**Description of symptoms**	**Date of medical advice**	**Precautions required**

First aid

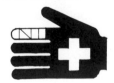

Emergency aid in the salon usually involves the treatment of minor accidental injuries. However, a qualified first aider would also be able to help with more serious injuries, such as bone fractures or heart attacks, before the patient is seen by a doctor.

* Full-size photocopiable versions of these forms appear on pages 242 and 243.

The aim of first aid is to prevent death or further damage to injured persons. If you have any doubt about an injury, always seek medical advice from a doctor or nurse at a health clinic or the casualty department at your local hospital.

A table of common accidents and conditions in the salon is shown below.

Common accidents and conditions in the salon

Accident/condition	Emergency procedure
Salon chemicals in the eye, e.g. perm lotions, bleaches, tints.	Wash the eye with running water (under the tap if possible). Continue applying water to the eye until medical assistance is available.
Salon chemicals on the skin, e.g. perm lotions, bleach.	Flood the area with water to dilute and remove the chemical.
Salon chemicals swallowed, e.g. chemicals placed in soft-drink containers and drunk by mistake.	Drink 2–3 glasses of water. Seek medical advice immediately.
Salon chemicals inhaled, e.g. strong bleach mixtures.	Move the person to fresh air immediately. Seek medical advice if coughing, choking or breathlessness lasts longer than 10–15 minutes.
Dry heat burns, e.g. from hairdriers, tongs, hot brushes, crimping irons.	Hold affected area under running cold water or apply ice pack (5–10 minutes). Seek medical advice if necessary.
Scalds, e.g. from hot water supplies or steamers.	Hold affected area under running cold water or apply ice pack (5–10 minutes). Seek medical advice if necessary.
Minor cuts.	Apply pressure until bleeding stops. Avoid direct contact with blood because of the risk of infectious diseases such as AIDS and Hepatitis B. Wherever possible, ask clients to use a clean piece of cotton wool and apply pressure themselves, then dispose of the cotton wool in a plastic bag or bin.
Severe cuts.	The blood flow from severe cuts should be stopped by applying pressure with either a clean towel or hands (covered with rubber gloves from the first aid box). Phone for an ambulance immediately.
Electric shock.	If someone is being electrocuted do not touch them as you will be electrocuted yourself. Turn off the electricity immediately, either by turning off the switches or pulling out the plug. If breathing has stopped then artificial respiration will need to be applied by a qualified first aider. Phone for an ambulance straight away.
Client distress, e.g. fainting.	This is caused by lack of oxygen to the brain. If someone feels faint, put their head between their knees and loosen any tight clothing. If the person has fainted, raise their legs on a cushion so that they are higher than the head.

Remember

RIDDOR states that all accidents must be reported in the accident register kept in the salon.

First aid kits

All salons should provide a **first aid box** (usually coloured green with a white cross) containing a first aid kit. It should include a list of contents, plus the following:

- A first aid guidance card

- Individually wrapped sterile adhesive dressings
- Medium, large and extra large sterile unmedicated dressings
- Sterile bandages (including a triangular bandage)
- Sterile eye pads, with attachment
- Scissors
- Tweezers
- Safety pins
- Antiseptic lotion

It is also advisable to keep disposable rubber or plastic gloves for dealing with wounds that are bleeding or weeping. Except in an emergency, aid should not be given without wearing these gloves because of the risk of AIDS and Hepatitis B.

To do

- Find out if your staff know where the first aid kit is located in your salon.
- Check the contents to see if anything is missing, or if there are any items which should not be there, e.g. medicines.

More serious signs of distress, such as heart attacks, stopped breathing, epileptic fits or fractures (from falls) should be dealt with by a qualified first aider. If you wish to qualify, contact your local St John's Ambulance Brigade who regularly run courses.

Test your knowledge

1 What is **emergency aid**?
2 When would a **qualified first aider** be needed?
3 When would you need to seek medical advice or **call an ambulance**?
4 What items would you expect to find in a **first aid box**?
5 State which colour codes of **fire extinguishers** can be used on:
   - electrical fires
   - non-electrical fires
   - and describe why this is important
6 If **perm lotion** accidentally ran into your client's eye, what would you do?
7 How would you deal with a child who has accidentally **swallowed** some **hydrogen peroxide**?
8 If some **bleach spills** on to your client's neck, how would you remove it?
9 What is the best treatment for someone who is **choking** after inhaling a strong chemical?
10 What could cause a **dry heat burn**?
11 How should you treat a **scald on the hand** from boiling water?
12 If you accidentally cut your client's ear, how should the **bleeding** be stopped?
13 Why must you always wear gloves when treating a person with **a severe cut**?
14 What is the most important action to take if someone is being **electrocuted**?
15 Why is it important to **raise a person's feet** if they have fainted?

Health and safety

The consequences of your failing to comply with Health and Safety requirements are serious. They include:

- Harming yourself, other staff or clients
- Notice being given by the Health and Safety Office for you to implement action
- Possible legal action

Non-compliance with Health and Safety requirements could be corrected by:

- Informing your manager or salon owner
- Correcting the compliance yourself if it is within your responsibility to do so
- Warning other people to avoid accidents whilst the matter is being dealt with

Routine health and safety checks

The following is a list of typical health and safety checks to be carried out in the salon:

Routine Health and Safety Checks*									
Inspection items/area	**Staff member responsible**	**Inspection dates/initials**							
Safety inspections									
Enforcing salon rules									
Inspecting electrical equipment									
First Aid kit									
Accident Book									
Fire exits /extinguishers /fire drills									
Day-to-day Health and Safety inspections									
COSHH assessments									

To do

- Find out exactly what your limits of authority are when dealing with non-compliance of Health and Safety regulations by your manager.

* A full-size photocopiable version of this form appears on page 244.

Security in the salon

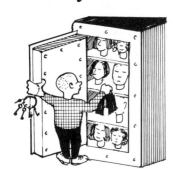

Security of people and possessions

The risk of theft or attack during business hours by salon visitors (such as clients, friends of other staff and business contacts) can be minimised if all your staff are trained to establish the identity of all salon callers. Most people will be able to give a valid reason for their visit.

If you approach someone who is acting suspiciously and they cannot give you a satisfactory reason for their visit, alert your manager or salon owner immediately. **Do not put yourself at any risk.** If the individual runs away, report the incident at once. It is likely that the police will need to be called and therefore you should document the facts. You will need to tell them clearly and accurately:

- The **date and time** of the incident
- **Where** the incident happened
- **What** actually took place
- **What** the intruder **looked like**

The police will also require **statements** from any other witnesses.

The **personal possessions** of both clients and staff also need protecting from theft. **Make sure that these are kept safely away from risk situations.** Clients' handbags, jewellery and any other valuables should

remain with them at all times. Valuable items or money belonging to staff should be securely stored during working hours, or kept with the individual, perhaps in their pockets.

Security of salon premises, fixtures and fittings

Salon premises are often very exposed to public view, having large windows and shop fronts. They should not be exposed to unnecessary risks. When closing the salon at night, take special care to ensure that:

- Doors, windows and cupboards are securely locked
- All money is removed from the till and stored in a safe
- No valuables are left in the salon
- All information or data relating to clients and staff is secure

Fixtures and fittings are usually identified by keeping an **inventory**. This is a comprehensive list and description of all the salon's furniture, fixtures and equipment.

Security of stock

Stock should always be available for use when required. If you notice any shortages, it may be because there is a thief on the premises.

If most stock is kept in a locked, secure area such as a storeroom, a cupboard or a retail cabinet, the opportunity for theft is minimised. It is a good idea to have a **key-holder** with the authority to dispense products, reducing the chance of theft even further.

Stock is a **valuable asset** belonging to the salon. If your salon has an accurate stock control system, it will be easier to spot discrepancies.

Unfortunately, theft by salon visitors is not the only way in which stealing occurs. Theft by staff (now often referred to as **shrinkage**) is another possibility. Theft of money, stock or equipment is an act of **gross misconduct**, and if discovered must be followed by disciplinary action, which may mean **instant dismissal**.

To prevent any misunderstanding, make sure that your staff understand your salon's policy in respect to purchasing salon stock.

Security of cash (and cash equivalents)

It is important to maintain a **safe and secure environment** at the reception area.

All monies must be secured, and products on display must be safeguarded. All personal details of clients, such as record systems, should be held under cover. If a client sees record cards lying around, she or he will have little confidence in the discretion of salon staff.

To keep reception secure, make sure that:

- The reception area is **staffed at all times**.
- All monies are kept securely in the till during the working day.
- The receptionist **never leaves the till drawer open** when it is not in use or if they have to leave the reception area for any reason.
- All **banknotes are checked** to ensure that both the metal strip and the watermark are present. On a forged note, either or both may be missing.

- When a client hands the receptionist a banknote, they place it **outside the till** until the receptionist has accurately counted the change.
- Money is **never left in the till overnight**.
- The till drawers are left **open but empty** at the end of the day to prevent a burglar from damaging them by forcing them open.
- Large amounts of money are **regularly transferred to a safe or bank**.
- Visits to the bank are **irregularly timed** to deter muggers. If the receptionist normally does the banking, someone else must be nominated to take over reception duties in the meantime. If possible, they should be accompanied.
- **Receipts** are given for all payments and bills retained.
- All bills, receipts and drawings or additions are noted so **the till balances**.
- At the end of the day, all monies are **checked, recorded and either secured in a safe or banked**.

Regular and random checks

You should take all possible preventative steps to minimise the risk of theft. Procedures should be set in place to **monitor till transactions, stock movements, and personal possessions**.

Money missing from the till will show up during the daily cashing up. Shortfalls will be noticed when the number of clients attended, services provided and retail stock items sold do not tally with the available money and cash equivalents, the till rolls and totals.

Missing items of stock will be noticed during normal stock control procedures, in routine situations where stock is not available as expected, and during spot checks and searches.

To do

- Make brief notes on your responsibilities and limits of authority for maintaining the security of your salon premises and contents.
- Describe how you would report any breaches of security to the relevant person.

Test your knowledge

1 List your own **responsibilities and limits of authority** in relation to your salon's **security systems**.
2 Describe how security is maintained in your salon in respect of:
   - People and possessions
   - Salon premises, fixtures and fittings
   - Stock
   - Cash and cash equivalents
3 Describe the two main potential **security problems** in a salon.
4 List what could happen if you **did not adhere to security procedures**.
5 How could you **correct** a potential security problem?
6 What constitutes a **breach of security**?
7 Describe a **salon policy** and **records** for dealing with **breaches of security**.

7 Artistic expression

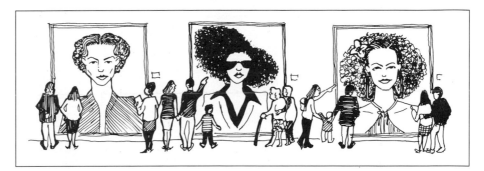

Creative thoughts

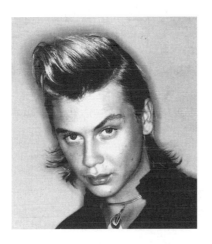
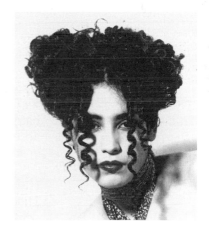

This chapter will focus on identifying and evaluating opportunities for creating images and developing those ideas.

Creative thoughts do not have to be completely original. They can be based on developing existing styles and ideas to create something slightly different. Many factors can spark creativity, including images from television and films, historical or artistic images, or pictures of film and pop stars.

Altering and modifying classic and fashion styles, adapting an avant-garde/alternative concept through creative use of colouring, perming and cutting techniques – these are just some ways in which hairdressers use artistic expression in their work.

To do
■ Put together a scrapbook of what you consider to be creative images, using pictures taken from magazines, fashion and history books, etc.

Creating images

There are many opportunities to be more creative with your work. They include hair and fashion shows, photographic sessions, special occasions such as weddings, or hairdressing competitions.

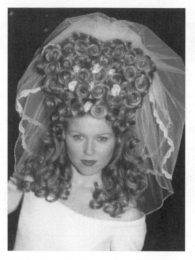 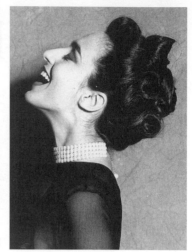

Hair and fashion shows

Hair shows provide many possibilities for creating artistic and creative images but require very detailed planing and preparation in order to be successful. Chapter 10 deals with a variety of promotional activities, including putting a hair show together (pages 163–170).

Special occasions

A classic example of a special occasion would be a wedding. Creating a hairstyle for a bride often involves working with **long hair** and **hair accessories**. There is often scope to transform the image of the client to create a total look which complements the wedding ensemble.

Hairdressing competitions

There are many categories of hairdressing competition, including **commercial**, **avant-garde** and **fantasy** styling. They give the hairdresser the opportunity to be highly creative, making use of strong colours and added hairpieces and creating a **total look** for the model, including **clothing, accessories and facial or body make-up**.

Photographic sessions

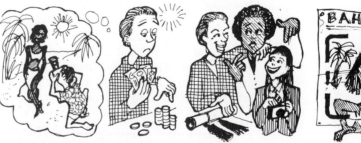 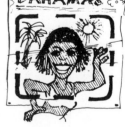

Producing a portfolio of your own work is a good way of promoting your hairdressing skills and creative talents to both existing and potential clients and employers. Photographs can also be submitted to hairdressing magazines for publication, which can help promote public recognition of your work.

Points to consider when planning a photo shoot

When planning a photo shoot remember to take the following into consideration:

- Budget constraints
- Photographer
- Models
- Location
- Backdrops
- Lighting

Budget constraints

These will influence the scale of your photo shoot. Does your budget allow you to hire a photographer, or will you be taking your own shots? Can you afford to pay for professional models or will you have to use clients or friends? Remember to set aside some of the budget for clothes, accessories, hairpieces, etc.

If you decide to use a professional photographer, choose someone who has experience of fashion and beauty photography. Looking through *Yellow Pages*, checking out **photo credits in trade journals and magazines** and contacting salons that produce their own photography are some ways of finding a photographer.

When interviewing photographers, always ask to see their **portfolios** and question them about work they have done for other salons/stylists.

Find out what the fees will be and whether they include **film and processing costs**, as these can often be additional. Some photographers have **assistants** who may be willing to do the work free, or at a reduced rate, in order to gain experience.

Models

If your budget allows, contact **model agencies** and explain the type of models you are looking for. Some model agencies can be reluctant to supply models if you wish to totally change their hair by cutting or colouring as this could affect any further modelling jobs. Models who are relatively new may be willing to pose free in return for shots to include in their own portfolios.

Whether you use professional models or find your own, always use **more than one model during a session**. You cannot predict how things will turn out and restricting yourself to one model could mean the shoot may not produce any good results. If using clients, friends or colleagues as models, remember the following:

- What someone looks like in 'real life' is no guide to how they will look on film. Some people can be extremely attractive yet photograph poorly. A good tip is to take a **Polaroid photo** before the actual session and assess the results.
- If you have someone with quite hard, but interesting features, try photographing them in **black and white**, which can soften the features.

Remember

The roles of colleagues involved in the photo session should be clearly defined and accurately communicated. See Chapter 1 on communication skills, and Chapter 14, pages 208–212.

- When choosing models, remember that the camera can make people appear heavier and larger than they are, so take time to choose models who are well proportioned.

Location

If you use a professional photographer, ask if they have a studio. If you prefer to work from your salon, check that this is OK with them. If you choose to take shots outdoors, remember that elaborate backgrounds and scenery can **detract from the subject** of your photographs.

If you use a location or have to go to the photographer's studio, remember to take all the **equipment and accessories** you will need with you. It is a good idea to **make a list in advance**.

Backdrops

When planning your photographs, think about where and how they will be used. Do you want to take head shots only or full frame? There are many types of backdrops that can be used: seamless paper and fabrics which will drape well are just two examples. Discuss colours and textures with your photographer.

Lighting

A professional photographer should be able to advise you on the most suitable lighting. This will vary depending on what you are showing – hair colour, shape, or texture. Do you prefer natural or artificial light? Are you taking colour, black and white shots, or both?

Developing your ideas

Once you have identified your opportunities for creating images, you must come up with, and develop, some specific ideas.

Ideas can come from many sources – hair and fashion magazines, brainstorming sessions with colleagues based around themes such as history, the 1970s, etc. Often the source will depend on the event or occasion, or the setting in which you want your work to be seen.

Once the ideas have been decided upon, they can be developed further. Remember that one idea can often spawn several others, and it is important to keep comprehensive, accurate and up-to-date records showing the planning, design and presentation of your ideas for future reference.

It is a good idea to compile a **portfolio** and include in it any plans, sketches, diagrams, illustrations and magazine cuttings. You can also include budget information, results of discussions and consultations with those involved, resources needed, such as equipment, materials – added hair, accessories, clothes, make-up and additional media requirements. It is also important to include information on where resources can be obtained – names and telephone numbers of suppliers and contacts, whether items have to be purchased or can be borrowed, perhaps those working on the idea with you have materials or equipment that could be used. Remember to record it all.

A **storyboard** showing the format of an idea and the preparation and resources required is also a good way of recording your ideas.

Remember
You will have set yourself a budget so try to stick to it, listing all resources – physical and material – and their costs. Don't forget to update this list as you go along – this is vital in order to keep within the allocated budget and prevent any unexpected costs.

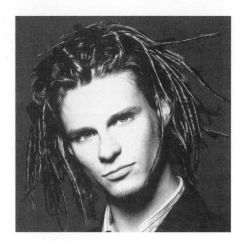

Adapting ideas

Remember that you can alter or modify your original ideas as required, depending on the opportunities selected.

- Try to create styles that can easily be transformed by **adding hairpieces or accessories**. This will save time and allow many different looks to be created without much effort.
- Try duplicating the same style on **different models** – this can often produce effective results.

Making your own hairpieces using **real or synthetic hair** is a cost-effective alternative to buying pre-prepared hairpieces. Hanks of real and synthetic hair can be purchased quite reasonably from wholesalers or by mail order, and both types of hair come in a variety of shades and tones which can be colour-matched to a model's natural hair.

Hair extensions can also be added to a model's hair to provide length and bulk, thus allowing a wider range of creative images to be produced (colour plate 7).

Trade magazines and exhibitions such as Salon International frequently promote suppliers of hair extension systems that use either synthetic or real hair.

Evaluating ideas

The suitability of the ideas chosen and their progression can be evaluated through discussion and consultation with colleagues. Look at what you have created and analyse its suitability. Are there any changes you need to make? Remember to encourage constructive comments and be willing to take on board what others involved in the project have to say.

Large-scale projects

When undertaking any large-scale projects it is important to consider:

- **Benefits to the salon.** These could include a **higher profile within the industry** and with the **general public**. This in turn could help to attract new staff, which might increase salon business and lead to further opportunities.

● **Benefits to you.** These could include **wider recognition of your own skills**, an **increase in your client base**, a **higher profile in the salon**, further job and career development and possible increase in salary.

Test your knowledge

1 Give examples of different forms of **artistic expression**.
2 Where could you find **inspiration** for **creating artistic images**?
3 Give examples of ways of coming up with **creative ideas**.
4 How could you **record your ideas** and their development?
5 List the **benefits to yourself and your salon** of promoting artistic images.
6 Where could you find information on **false hair/hair extensions**?
7 List the things you need to consider when planning a **photo shoot.**
8 Give examples of **forms of evaluation** that can be used
9 Why is it important to **set and work to a budget**?

8 African/Afro-Caribbean hair

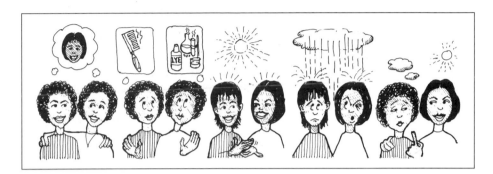

Characteristics of African/Afro-Caribbean hair

Natural tight-curly African/Afro-Caribbean hair can be quite difficult to manage as it has a tendency to tangle and become very dry. However, once it is straightened by either temporary or permanent means, it becomes extremely manageable and easy to style.

If you can offer services to African/Afro-Caribbean clients such as relaxing, curly perms using heated equipment, conditioning (often called 'steaming' as the steamer is used to help conditioners to penetrate the hair), cutting, hair extensions and 'weave-on's', then your salon's professional image will be enhanced. You will also gain all the benefits of a greatly increased clientele.

African/Afro-Caribbean hair structure

This hair is naturally dark because it contains more **melanin**.

It also needs more care and conditioning than Caucasian (European) hair because of its curly and crinkly shape. It tends to tangle easily, and may be damaged and break at the ends simply by being disentangled with combs and brushes.

Its curl is formed because of **uneven keratinisation**. This means that the keratin in the hair is more dense on the inside of the curl or wave – the 'para' cortex – and less dense on the outside of the curl or wave – the 'ortho' cortex.

African/Afro-Caribbean hair may be:

- **Tight-curly.** If you look at the roots of the hair, you will see that it springs back curly near the scalp. Generally, tight-curly hair takes relaxer more easily.

131

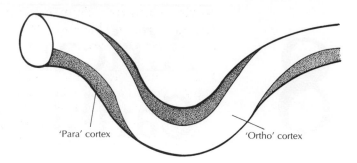

'Para' cortex   'Ortho' cortex

African/Afro-Caribbean hair structure

- **Wavy.** If the hair is wavy at the roots, then it is generally stronger and needs a stronger relaxer.
- **Straight.** Ask the client if she has had a **relaxer** (a permanent straightener) or whether her hair has been **pressed** (a temporary relaxer).

To do
■ Re-read Chapter 1 regarding: – The texture of hair – Establishing hair condition (porosity, elasticity) – Hair structure, particularly the hair's cuticle, cortex and temporary and permanent bonds

African/Afro-Caribbean hair has slightly more cuticle layers than Caucasian hair and is therefore initially more resistant to chemical processes such as tinting, bleaching, perming and relaxing. Because it has more cuticle it has less volume of cortex. This means that once chemicals have entered through the cuticle and into the cortex they will process African/Afro-Caribbean hair more quickly than Caucasian hair.

Health and safety

Make sure your client is correctly protected during thermal styling and relaxing by using the correct products, tools and equipment in accordance with the manufacturer's instructions, salon requirements and local bye-laws. During consultations when you are examining the hair and scalp check for infections and infestations to reduce the risk of infecting either yourself or others in the salon.

Keeping your work area clean and tidy minimises the risk of cross infection, maintains a professional salon image and allows you to work efficiently without disrupting other staff who may be working nearby.

Remember to check all of your electrical equipment before you use it for possible damage, loose connections and an up-to-date electrical safety test label to minimise the risk of accidents.

The Cosmetic Products (Safety) Regulations 1989

These cover the rules that recommend different volumes and strengths of hydroxide-based products – i.e. hydrogen peroxide (which is mixed with tints and bleaches and an ingredient in some perm neutralisers) and relaxers which are sodium, calcium and potassium hydroxide. Product strengths will vary between those made for professional and non-professional (i.e. retail) use.

You can check the product strengths from the manufacturer's instructions and guidance notes. Further guidance can also be obtained by contacting the individual manufacturer or by contacting the Hairdressing Manufacturers & Wholesalers Association (HMWA) at 25 West Street, Haslemere, Surrey, GU27 2AP, tel. 01428 654336.

Styling African/Afro-Caribbean hair with heated equipment

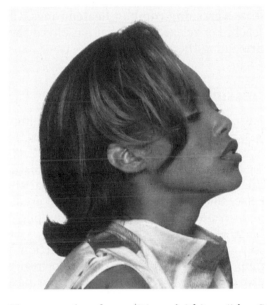

Temporarily straightened hair

Shampooed and conditioned African/Afro-Caribbean hair may be blow-dried and temporarily straightened by using a **wide-toothed comb hand-dryer attachment**.

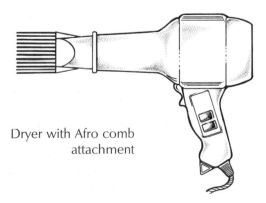

Dryer with Afro comb attachment

Wet hair can also be wrap set with a suitable blow-dry lotion/wrapping lotion or mousse to achieve straightness. Three rollers are placed in a downwards direction at the crown area, the hair is parted at the front (off-centre), then brushed smoothly flat around the head then dried under a hood dryer.

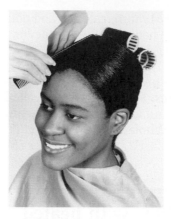
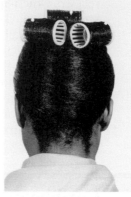
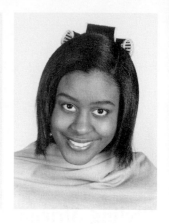

Once the virgin hair is straight it can be moulded into shape by using either a **pressing comb** or **heated tongs**. **Chemically treated** (coloured, bleached or relaxed hair) that has already been processed needs **greater care** during thermal styling.

Pressing combs

Hair pressing or thermal hair straightening is a **temporary process**. It breaks the hydrogen bonds by using heat and tension.

The hair's natural **water content** or **moisture** is lost during this process, which is why **pressing oils** and **thermal styling** sprays are used to help replace this moisture. These oil-based products form a protective layer over the hair and may contain silicones or long-chain hydrocarbons.

They are sprayed evenly onto each section of dry hair before pressing begins. Protective moisturising scalp creams may also be used to prevent scalp dryness and are applied with the fingers section by section before hair pressing.

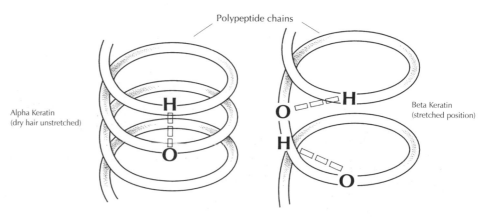

Alpha and beta keratin

Tight-curly hair in its unstretched state is described as being in **alpha keratin**. When the hair has been stretched straight by using heated styling equipment, it is in a **beta keratin** state.

Once the hair is dampened again, either by shampooing or through the client perspiring or being caught in the rain, then the hair will revert to its natural curly **alpha keratin** state again.

Regular or non-electric combs

These combs are made of steel or brass with a wooden handle. They are heated by small electric heaters or gas stoves. Eight sizes are available, the space between the teeth varying – small teeth are used for fine hair, large teeth for coarse hair. Remember, the **smaller** the teeth, the more **tension**, which will create a **straighter effect**.

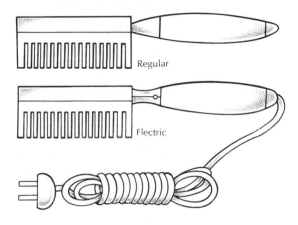

Pressing combs

Thermostatically controlled combs

These have a set working temperature.

Soft pressing

Before proceeding, always check the scalp for soreness caused by chemical treatments or scratches (from previous pressing or styling). **Do not continue** if this is the case, but recommend **conditioning treatments**.

Using the following method, 70% of the curl can be removed.

Method

● Shampoo, condition and dry the hair.

● Apply a suitable **pressing oil, thermal styling spray, pomade or cream** to the hair and scalp to protect against scorching and add sheen.

● Take **sections of 1.25 cm** ($\frac{1}{2}$ in.), starting at the back and holding the hair at **90° to the head**. Check the heat of the comb, then insert it **1.25 cm from the scalp**.

● Slide the comb down the hair mesh, turning it over so that the **back of the comb** creates tension and straightens the hair.

● **Comb each mesh** of hair **two or three times** and gradually work towards the front.

● Once **complete**, apply a dressing cream, brush it through and style with curling tongs.

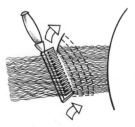

Inserting a pressing comb

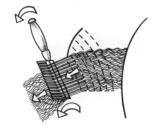

Pulling hair straight using the back of a pressing comb

Hard pressing

This method removes almost all of the curl but is more damaging to the hair than soft pressing. Simply **repeat the soft pressing method** or straighten the hair again with **Marcel thermal waving irons**. These non-electric irons are slid down the hair mesh, pulling it straight.

Cleaning pressing combs

Always wipe the pressing comb free of grease and loose hairs after use. Clean combs work better, so use a commercially prepared product regularly to remove carbon build-up.

Thermal styling

Remember

Always use a thermal styling spray before tonging to protect the hair from the heat of the tongs.

Tongs can be used to produce a variety of effects, from curls and waves to ringlets or just for curling the ends of the hair (as in a bob). They are often used after blow drying the hair straight. Hot brushes and heated rollers can also be used to thermally style African/Afro-Caribbean hair.

Many stylists who work with African/Afro-Caribbean hair prefer to use tongs that are heated up in a separate heater because several sizes are available at the same time to give a variety of styles and effects.

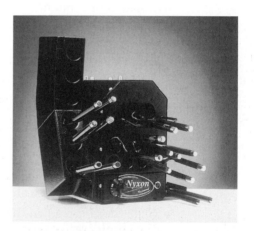

Afro tongs

Method for using tongs

The two movements used when tonging are

- **Opening and closing the tongs** – which allows the tongs to move through the hair
- **Turning the tongs** – which curls the hair

It is a combination of these two movements which can give the following effects:

- Waves
- Barrel curls or root curls
- Spiral curls
- Off base or end curls

Remember

The treatment for burns from hot electrical equipment is to hold the affected area under running cold water, or apply an ice-pack for at least 10 minutes.

Remember

Do not hard press (with a pressing comb) or repeat the use of non-electric tongs on chemically treated (i.e. relaxed) hair.

Always smooth the hair first by placing the tongs at the roots, gripping the hair, then sliding down the hair mesh a few times. This both smoothes the cuticle and allows you to establish a firm grip on the hair with the tongs.

Problems associated with thermal styling

Burns

- **Burns of the hair.** Remember always to use a **lower temperature** on fine, bleached, tinted and chemically treated hair.
- **Burns of the scalp or skin.** Always check the temperature of the irons on either a white tissue or a white towel. If it scorches or leaves a brown mark, allow the equipment to cool down before use.

Traction alopecia

Excessive **tension** used when hot-pressing hair by pulling at the hair shaft can lead to **hair breakage or loosening** of the hair in the follicle, causing traction alopecia. This baldness can become permanent if traction or pulling is carried out over a long period.

Cicatrical alopecia

This is a **permanent bald patch** where the hair follicles have been destroyed. It can be due to **scarring** from a heat burn, from **thermal styling** or even from a **strong chemical relaxer** left on the scalp for too long.

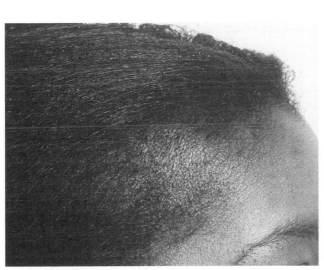

Traction alopecia

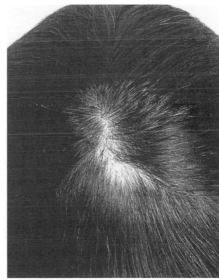

Cicatrical alopecia

Thermal styling difficulties and corrections

Difficulty	Correction
Hair scorched.	Recheck the tool temperature before use on white tissue.
Very short hair.	Use thermal oil spray on the scalp and avoid touching the scalp with heated equipment.
Possible hair breakage.	Cut the hair if possible, advise deep conditioning treatments to add moisture and protein before continuing.

Electric tongs

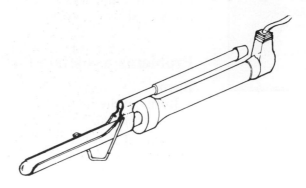

Precautions when using tongs
- Always pick them up by their **handles**.
- Always place a **comb** between hot tongs and the client's scalp when you are working near the scalp.
- Always use the **stand** or **rest** attached to the tongs to prevent work surfaces from becoming scorched, and plastic surfaces (such as equipment trolleys) from becoming melted.
- Never put hot tongs into your tool bag. Allow them to **cool** first.
- Remember to **switch the tongs off** as soon as you have finished using them – it helps to prevent accidents.
- Light-coloured hair can be **discoloured** and **scorched** by the tongs, so do not have them **too hot** or use them for **too long** on the hair.
- Flexes can become twisted and insulation can gradually wear away, making the tool dangerous. **Flexes must be checked regularly.**

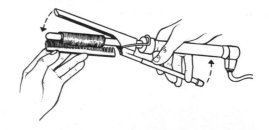

Using electric tongs

Relaxing

Relaxers are very popular with clients who have excessively curly or wavy hair because once their hair is permanently straightened they have a much wider choice of hairstyles. It also takes the pain out of combing their hair.

Relaxers may be applied

- To virgin hair
- To the regrowth of previously relaxed hair
- To correct an uneven result from a previous relaxing treatment

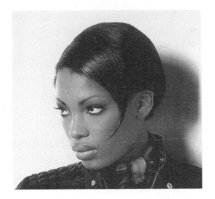

Relaxed hair

> **Remember**
>
> Products must be stored, used and disposed of according to the manufacturer's instructions.

Tight-curly African/Afro-Caribbean hair has more cuticle scales and is initially more difficult to chemically process.

Relaxing creams are extremely **alkaline**, with a pH of 10–14, which means they are very strong chemicals. **Sodium hydroxide relaxers** (caustic soda, sometimes called **lye**) are the strongest and fastest-acting chemicals.

Calcium hydroxide (occasionally **potassium hydroxide** or **guanidine hydroxide**) relaxers (sometimes called **no-lye**) are not as strong, but are gentler on the scalp and tend to lighten the colour, causing a reddish tinge. They are not as effective as other relaxers and do not require the scalp to be based. These relaxers are often available for home use, but leave the hair dry and brittle.

> **Remember**
>
> If **too many cystine bonds** are broken by the relaxer being left on too long the hair will become weak and break.

Both of these straightening chemicals permanently change the structure of the hair by changing one-third of the **cystine** bonds into new **lanthionine** bonds (with one sulphur atom), which keep the hair straight. This process (sometimes known as **hydrolysis**) is **stopped** by a **neutralising shampoo**. The low pH of this shampoo stops any further chemical action.

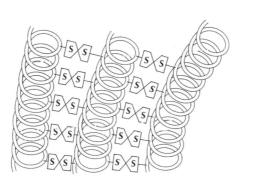

Tight curly/wavy hair with disulphide bonds intact

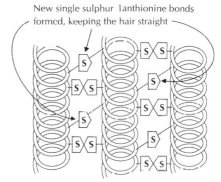

New single sulphur lanthionine bonds formed, keeping the hair straight

After being shaped with relaxing cream, processed and neutralising shampoo applied

Neutralising shampoos for relaxers

Shampoo the hair thoroughly to remove excess relaxer from the hair and scalp and stop the action of the relaxer.

Remember

Neutralising shampoos work differently from perm neutralisers.

Never use a neutralising shampoo after a normal perm, or a perm neutraliser after straightening hair.

On the **second shampoo**, some manufacturers recommend firmly combing the hair straight – but remember to be gentle on the scalp.

Leave for **five minutes**, then rinse thoroughly.

Check the manufacturer's instructions: some products change colour to show that the neutralising is complete.

Blot the hair, then use a **pH-balanced moisturising conditioner** (to restore the hair to its normal acidic level) as a treatment and leave for ten minutes, then **rinse thoroughly**.

Examining the hair and scalp

To do

■ Re-read the sections in Chapter 1 on strand tests, elasticity tests, porosity tests and incompatibility tests (pages 25–27).

Remember

Relax only the regrowth area of bleached, highlighted or permanently coloured hair to avoid hair breakage from over processing.

Remember

The scalp is very sensitive after either cane row or extensions have been removed. Do not chemically relax hair on the same day that they are removed.

Always recommend a reconditioning treatment and allow two weeks before applying a relaxer to allow the hair's elasticity to return, and the scalp's sensitivity to return to normal.

1 Check the client's scalp for any **soreness, cuts, abrasions or disorders**. If in doubt, do not proceed. If the client has an **itchy or flaky scalp**, then it is likely to be **sensitive** and may need a **no-lye relaxer**. Clients with a **build-up of shampoo and conditioning products** on their hair should have their hair **shampooed five days before** a relaxing treatment. Leave 72 hours between tinting/bleaching and relaxing treatments.
2 Check the client's hair condition for:
   ● **Elasticity and tensile strength** (elasticity test)
   ● **Tightness of curl** (strand test, i.e. product strength and timing)
   ● **Texture and porosity** (porosity test)
   ● **Previous chemical processes** (incompatibility test)
   ● Any **breakage** (elasticity test)
   If you are in any doubt, proceed with the necessary test and suggest some reconditioning treatments.
3 Check the client's record card for any previous treatments.
4 Check exactly what degree of straightness the client requires (use photographs from style books)

Matching relaxer to hair type

Relaxers are **very strong chemicals**.

● Make sure that you have sufficient product knowledge before using them. Try writing out the manufacturers' instructions in your own words.
● Make sure that you are using the **correct straightening chemical** for the hair, and the **correct strength** of chemical.

Sodium hydroxide (lye) relaxers

Nowadays these are oil based and leave the hair with body and shine. Look at the amount of curl in the hair by parting it – the more resistant curl formation is an important factor when choosing strengths of a relaxer. For example, coarse, tight-curly, virgin hair may need a super relaxer – normal curly hair may need a regular relaxer.

A choice of strengths is available (with a pH range of 12–13):

- For **fine**, **tinted** or **lightened** hair (hair that has been previously chemically treated) use **mild relaxers**
- For **normal**, **medium-textured** hair use **regular relaxers**
- For **coarse** hair use **strong** or **super-relaxers**

Calcium hydroxide (no-lye) relaxers

No-lye relaxers may not necessarily be calcium hydroxide: sometimes the chemical is potassium, guanidine or lithium hydroxide.

Calcium hydroxide relaxers are more suitable for clients with a **sensitive scalp** because they are **not as strong** as sodium hydroxide (lye) relaxers. This is the reason why no-lye relaxers are more often available for retail use.

Calcium hydroxide (no-lye) relaxers are mixed with an activator, and once mixed must not be used after 12 hours.

These relaxers **need more manipulation** and smoothing straight during development and often need the application of heat.

To do

- Take cuttings of tight-curly and wavy hair and strand-test them with a sodium hydroxide and calcium hydroxide relaxer. Make a note of the development times and any differences in the elasticity and condition of the hair.

To base or not to base?

Always read the **manufacturer's instructions** regarding basing the scalp. Most **sodium hydroxide** relaxers do **need a protective basing cream**.

If the client has a sensitive scalp you should choose a **calcium hydroxide (no-lye) relaxer**, which **does not require a protective basing cream**.

Protection of the client and hairdresser

- **Always** wear rubber gloves, and gown up your client properly.
- **Protect** the client's hairline and scalp by applying protective base (or Vaseline) or special basing cream.
- **Do not shampoo the hair or brush the scalp.** If the scalp is sensitive apply protective basing cream (or Vaseline) to the scalp area section by section (like a tint). **Place the cream,** do not press or rub it in, as **it must not cover the hair.**
- Check the **manufacturer's instructions**. If a pre-relaxer treatment (filler) needs to be used, apply it evenly at this stage and blot off any excess.
- If the relaxer accidentally enters the eye **it could cause blindness**, so shield the unaffected eye with one hand, and **flush the affected eye** with lots of water. Seek medical help if the irritation persists. If the product comes into contact with the client's skin or clothes, flush the area immediately to dilute and remove the chemical.
- Always try to work in a **ventilated area** so that the fumes are less hazardous to both you and the client. You are responsible.

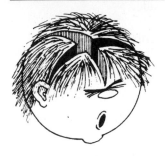

Application methods

Section the hair into four and then prepare to apply the relaxer to the border of each section, leaving the hairline until last ('hot cross bun' technique).

Start at the crown area of section 1, take small sections and apply relaxer cream with the back of the comb or a brush, 6 mm from the scalp area to allow for product expansion. Work your way down to the nape. Complete sections 1 and 2 at the back, then complete sections 3 and 4 at the front, working **towards the front hairline**. Apply to the front hairline, where the hair is more porous, last.

Smooth the hair straight with your gloved hand to spread the product. **Cross-check the application** in the opposite direction, reapplying relaxer to any uncovered areas. The product will swell during development.

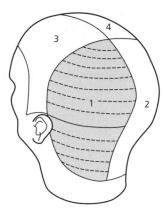

Remember that on virgin hair the relaxer needs to be applied to the lengths and ends first then to the root area once the processing has started, so that the roots do not take too quickly because of body heat.

Regrowth applications

With previously straightened hair, apply to the regrowth only, taking care not to overlap onto the previously straightened hair.

Development and processing

Leave the hair as straight as possible. Do not continually comb the hair – it may easily break and lose its tensile strength.

Develop the product according to the manufacturer's instructions. This may take anything from 2 to 18 minutes. Check it continually by removing some of the product from a strand (strand test) and letting the hair relax with your comb to see the degree of straightness.

When processing is complete, **rinse at a back wash basin with a strong stream of warm water**. Start at the hairline and let the force of the water remove the cream. Do not use your hands. Rinse until the water runs clear. Some manufacturers advise the use of a reconstructor at this stage, which should be left on for five minutes before the **neutralising shampoo** is applied.

Problems and corrections

Overprocessing

If the product touches the scalp or skin for a prolonged period it will cause **serious irritation, burning and damage**. If the client complains that her skin or scalp are 'burning', **rinse the relaxer off immediately** and use the neutralising shampoo.

If the product **stays in contact with the hair for too long**, the hair may **become brittle, break off or even dissolve**. Do not relax the hair if you think there will be any hair breakage.

Never use any **additional heat** (from hairdryers or accelerators or steamers) when processing sodium hydroxide relaxers – they develop very quickly and could dissolve the hair.

Corrections regarding processing

Overprocessed hair will need a course of **reconditioning treatments** or **restructurants**. Do not attempt to re-process the hair – it is best kept regularly trimmed until the chemically treated hair has grown out.

If the skin or scalp is **irritated** then, after flushing with water, apply a **soothing moisturising cream** to the area.

Underprocessing

If the relaxing product used was **not strong enough**, if it were **incorrectly applied**, resulting in roots, mid lengths or ends being omitted, or if it was **removed too soon**, then the hair will still look **crinkly** and **frizzy**, resulting in different degrees of movement.

After leaving sufficient time between relaxing and the corrective treatment (1–2 weeks) a suitable strength relaxer may be applied to the **underprocessed** areas of the hair (isolate the rest of the hair with a protective product).

The hair is then developed and the neutralising shampoo applied as normal to achieve perfectly relaxed hair that looks both straight and shiny.

Corrections regarding products

If a **sodium hydroxide (lye)** relaxer was used, then a **weaker strength** product may be reapplied to the underprocessed areas. Take **great care** with the application and constantly **check the development**.

If a **calcium hydroxide (no-lye)** relaxer has been used, which is a weaker chemical than the sodium hydroxide (lye), it may be that you did not check that the client's **shampoos** and **conditioning products** were removed from the hair beforehand. Remember that calcium hydroxide (no-lye) relaxers tend to make the hair feel hard and clients are more likely to overuse conditioning products as a result.

It is possible to re-relax a no-lye treatment in the same way as a lye relaxer, but remember that calcium hydroxide relaxers can make the hair red. Reapplication of the product may increase this redness.

Remember

Always allow sufficient time between relaxing and corrective treatments to minimise any damage to the hair.

Remember

Poor-conditioned hair is **better set** than blow dried after relaxing.

Remember

Never apply a sodium hydroxide (lye) relaxer over a calcium hydroxide (no-lye) relaxer in an attempt to re-process the hair. The no-lye relaxer deposits calcium in the hair and would act as a barrier.

Record cards

Always keep your records up to date.

Relaxer Record Card

Client name	Address	Daytime telephone number
_____	_____	_____

Date of 1st relaxer _____	Date _____	Special notes _____
Colour treated/natural _____	Make of relaxer _____	_____
If treated, product used _____	Product strength _____	Neutralising time & method _____
Texture _____	Virgin head or regrowth _____	Conditioner _____
Condition _____	Result required _____	Result obtained _____
_____	Development time & method _____	Stylist _____

Other African/Afro-Caribbean hair styling products

African/Afro-Caribbean hair has a natural tendency to dryness, and when it is either thermally styled or chemically processed it needs a full range of conditioning products.

Shampoos

Shampoos for African/Afro-Caribbean hair contain both **mild detergents** and a higher concentration of **moisturising and detangling agents, creams and oils**.

Deep-acting conditioners

These are often **oil based**, adding **moisture** to the hair, and contain **protein** and **polymer** formulations to strengthen the hair. They must be left on for a minimum of three minutes, but most **benefit by the addition of heat** (either from a steamer or by covering with a plastic cap and placing under a dryer).

Reconstructors

These help to **replace proteins, amino acids and oils**. They are sometimes used after the relaxer is rinsed off and before the neutralising shampoo is applied.

Moisturisers

These are sprayed onto **wet hair** to add moisture and body to the hair and to keep it wet during cutting.

Oil sheen sprays

These are used in the same way as thermal styling sprays on **dry hair** to give extra shine and finish.

Spritz, holding sprays and gels

These are all used for a finishing **final hold** on the hair.

Test your knowledge

1 Describe the following **health and safety** considerations:
   - Client preparation
   - Use of personal protective equipment
   - Cross-infections and infestations
   - Electrical equipment checks
2 Why does African/Afro-Caribbean hair need **more care and conditioning** than Caucasian hair?
3 Sketch and label a diagram to show **afro hair structure**.
4 Which **bonds** in the cortex are broken by **thermal styling**?
5 Describe the **equipment** needed to **thermally style hair**.
6 What happens to the **water in the hair during thermal styling**?
7 How should you **test the temperature** of thermal styling equipment?
8 What could happen if you **failed to test the temperature** of thermal styling equipment?
9 Describe the **products needed** to keep the hair and scalp in good condition **during thermal styling** and how to use them.
10 Describe the reasons why **soft pressing** is more suitable for chemically treated hair and hard pressing is more suitable for virgin hair.
11 Describe how to **prevent burns** to:
   - the hair
   - the scalp or skin
   during thermal styling.
12 Describe **traction alopecia** and its causes.
13 Describe **cicatrical alopecia** and its causes.
14 Describe three potentially difficult **problems** which may occur during **thermal styling** and how you could correct them.
15 Which **bonds** in the cortex are broken by **chemical relaxing**?
16 Name the **new bonds** that are formed during the relaxing process.
17 Why is a **neutralising shampoo** used after relaxing?
18 Why is it not possible to **perm** relaxed hair?
19 What should you look for when examining the **scalp before relaxing**?
20 Describe the differences between **sodium hydroxide (lye)** relaxers and **calcium hydroxide (no-lye)** relaxers. How you would choose to use each?
21 Describe the **three main types** of sodium hydroxide (lye) relaxers.
22 Which type of relaxer needs a **basing cream**?
23 How should you **protect your client** before relaxing?
24 How should you **protect yourself** before applying a relaxer?
25 How does the **COSHH Act** relate to using relaxing chemicals?
26 During the application of relaxers describe how to:
   - **Section** the hair
   - **Apply** the product to **virgin hair**
   - **Apply** the product to a **regrowth**
   - **Cross-check** the application
   - **Develop** the product
   - Take a **strand test**
   - **Remove** the product from the hair
   - Use a **neutralising shampoo**
27 What could happen to the hair and scalp/skin if the relaxer is **overprocessed**, and why?
28 How could you **rectify** overprocessed hair?
29 What does the hair look like if it is **underprocessed**?

continued

Test your knowledge *continued*

30 If a sodium hydroxide (lye) relaxer was **underdeveloped** resulting in different degrees of movement, how could you **correct** it?

31 Why should you allow **sufficient time** to elapse between relaxing and a corrective type of treatment?

32 **Why** could a calcium hydroxide (no-lye) relaxer be **underdeveloped**?

33 Why must you take **greater care** when correcting an underdeveloped calcium hydroxide (no-lye) relaxer?

34 What effect do **different temperatures** have on the relaxing process?

35 Why can you **not correct** a calcium hydroxide (no-lye) relaxer with a sodium hydroxide (lye) relaxer?

36 Why is a pH-balanced **moisturising conditioner** used after relaxing?

9 Creative setting

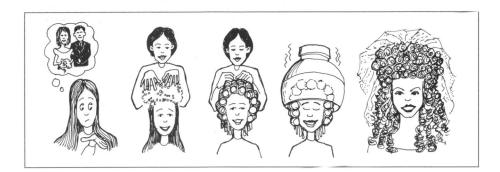

Modern setting

Traditionally, setting was reserved for older clients in the salon. However, with the introduction of Velcro rollers and Molton Browners, both of which produce more modern casual, unstructured looks, setting has once again become popular. Heated rollers are also enjoying a revival.

Modern styles of setting can be divided into three groups:

- Classic
- Fashion
- Alternative

Classic styles

Classic styles have timeless appeal and include dressing the hair up into **French pleats**, **chignons** and **rolls**, with longer hair being worn down in **waves** or **smoothed under**. Shorter hair can be **pin-curled** or **finger-waved** to create movement.

Fashion styles

Fashion styles are styles that are currently 'in vogue'. Setting longer hair on Molton Browners will give **spiral** or **corkscrew-type curls**, which can

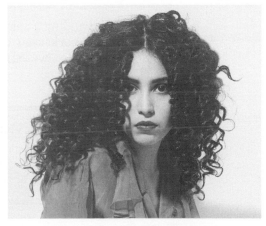

be separated and defined using **wax**. Putting in Velcro rollers using traditional methods of rollering to create volume and curl will produce soft, casual, yet fashionable styles on short, medium or long hair. Changing the **set**, or **pli**, **direction** can create many variations on one head. When **putting hair up** modern styling looks towards a **sleeker, flatter finish** with a focal point of height or volume with very little root lift in the crown area.

Many-strand **plaits** or **braids** can be worn up, down, or across the head and can be woven under or over to create different looks. Once the basic skills of braiding have been learned, there are many different results that can be created using variations on the same theme.

Both classic and fashion techniques of dressing hair up are very popular for special occasions such as weddings. Bridal styles often incorporate ornamentation such as fresh or synthetic flowers in the final dressing.

Alternative styles

These are the more **outrageous** and **creative high-fashion designs**, often incorporating **ornamentation** and **added hairpieces**. They are usually restricted to **competition**, **photographic** and **show work**. Usually the style has some basis in classic or fashion styles, but with the details exaggerated to create more dramatic results (colour plate 7).

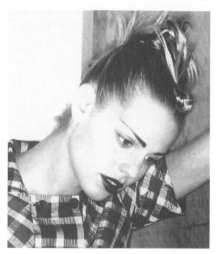 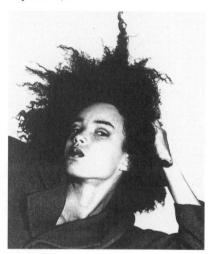

To do

■ List the setting and dressing services offered in your salon and the time allocated for each when booking appointments.

For example, winding a spiral set using **chopsticks** will produce very dramatic, **tight corkscrew curls** and synthetic hair can be used when dressing hair up to give extra height and bulk, enabling very exaggerated results to be produced.

To do

■ Using style magazines, collect examples of classic, alternative and fashion styles and consider how you would recreate each one, listing products, tools, equipment and techniques you would use.
■ Read Chapter 1, page 6, on how to keep up to date with fashion trends.

Client consultation

- Use your **style book** to discuss the style with your client and select the type of style suitable.
- Discuss the **occasion** with your client. Wedding or evening function?
- Discuss the **clothes** your client will be wearing. Do they have a high or low neckline? Will the hairstyle balance with the clothes?
- **How much time will you need** to dress the style? Dressing hair up will take longer.
- Discuss the **cost** with the client. Many salons charge extra for putting hair up.

General points to consider when deciding on a style include:

- **The shape of the head.** If it is flat at the back more hair will be needed there to balance it.
- **The shape of the face.** A round or square face can be softened by a few tendrils of hair around the face.
- **The amount of hair.** If dressing hair up, does the client have enough hair or will a hairpiece be needed?
- **Hair structure.** If the hair is very straight it will need setting first. If very curly, it may need to be straightened.
- **Hair texture.** Frizzy hair may need wax or dressing cream to smooth it. Strong, coarse hair may need a strong styling lotion for control.
- **Hair length.** The longer the hair, the heavier it becomes. This can create problems when dressing hair up.

When putting long hair up, in addition to looking at the hair we also need to consider the following:

- What is the **occasion**? Is the client going to a special event – ball/wedding etc.?
- **What will the client be wearing?** If the outfit has a low neckline, leave a few tendrils of hair hanging down – having all the hair pinned up can make the client feel bare.
- Is the outfit **ornate** or **plain/sleek**? Ornate dress with very fussy hair may look over-done – preferably keep the style simple and chic/classic. If the dress is plain then go for a more adventurous/creative hairstyle.
- Will there be a **head-dress** or hair **ornamentation**? If the headwear is very ornate, keep the style simple and uncluttered.
- Don't forget **shoes** – high shoes with high hairstyles could make the client look very tall (remember, the style should look balanced and in proportion).
- Does the client have a male **escort/partner** for the event? You'll need to consider his height – creating a 'structure' that will tower over the partner will not be pleasing to the eye, or the couple concerned!

Preparation of client

Gown the client using gown and towel to protect clothing.

If the hair is being dressed up, advise the client to wear **a top that does not have to be pulled off over the head** as this will spoil the hairstyle – a blouse/top with buttons is best.

Consider **hair preparation** – does the hair need to be freshly washed? If not, ask the client to wash her hair before coming in if possible. Do you really need to set the head on traditional rollers before putting it up? This can sometimes create too much root movement (and also roller marks that are hard to disguise) – heated rollers are ideal for creating curl at the ends of the hair without too much root lift.

Bridal hair

If you do a lot of bridal hair, consider putting together a bridal package. This should include a thorough consultation, rehearsal session plus an appointment for the final date with a total price given for the package. A nice touch is to also include champagne on the morning of the wedding. For the rehearsal session you will need the head-dress and veil, and ask the client to wear something white and plain to enhance the head-dress – alternatively, keep some white and cream fabric at the salon to use. Get her to wear her wedding make-up so that a true image of the actual look can be achieved. Taking Polaroid pictures of the finished style will help when it comes to recreating the style on the wedding day and will remind the bride-to-be of what she will look like. Some salons offer make-up and manicure services; these could also be included in the bridal package.

Remember: whatever the occasion – always allocate enough time to create the look without having to rush. A practice session is a good idea as it allows you to try out a variety of different styles before the actual event and gives your client the opportunity to say how she feels – and to change her mind if necessary.

Client satisfaction

To ensure client satisfaction, it is essential that clients are happy not only with their hairstyle but also with the **hair care advice** and the general treatment they receive whilst in the salon. Before commencing any service, a thorough consultation should be carried out leading to a discussion on the style required. Combined with the practical skills of the stylist, this should ensure that clients are happy with the service they receive.

Remember

The client is the most important person in the salon. If a client is not satisfied with the service they receive they will not return. A happy client will return to the salon for further treatments.

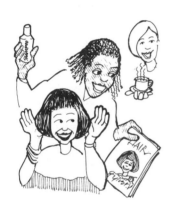

To do

■ Re-read Chapter 1 on client consultation and feedback on services provided.

Tools, equipment and products used in setting

Whether you are creating a classic, fashion or alternative style, selecting the correct tools, equipment and products is essential if the finished result is to be successfully achieved.

Brushes

These are used before setting to disentangle the hair during consultation and after setting to remove the roller marks and dress the hair.

Flat brushes with open tufts or bristles are normally used as these do not get tangled in the hair.

Combs

Tail combs have plastic or metal tails and are used for sectioning the hair when inserting rollers.

Dressing-out combs can have larger teeth for disentangling hair and fine teeth which are useful for back-combing.

Traditional rollers

These can be smooth or spiky. Spiky rollers are better for holding hair in place but can be difficult to keep clean and free from hairs, often becoming tangled in longer hair. Smooth setting rollers are more suitable for use on highly bleached or porous hair and when setting hair for competition or photographic work, as they do not leave ridges or marks on the hair.

Rollers are available in cylindrical and conical shapes.

Velcro rollers

Velcro rollers, designed for use on dry hair, have small hooks which grip the hair as it is being wound, enabling them to remain secured in the hair without the need for pins.

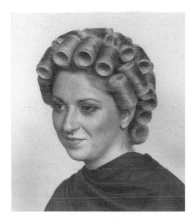

Heated rollers

These rollers are pre-heated and wound into dry hair, secured and left to cool down before removing. They are ideal for giving a quick foundation curl when putting hair up.

Remember
Excessive use of heat and heated styling equipment can cause damage to the hair and in some cases to the scalp if care is not taken. When using heated rollers, wrap tissue paper around rollers or ends of hair before winding to diffuse heat and prevent excessive damage to hair.

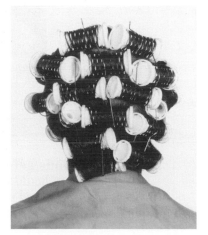

Molton Browners

These come in **foam** or **rubber** and are used to give a spiral or corkscrew/ringlet effect on long hair. They will produce a curl result which is even along the hairs' length.

As with conventional setting, whichever type of curler is used, the size will determine the end result, with **larger** rollers producing **soft results** and **smaller** ones giving **tighter curls**.

Pins and clips

Straight pins are used to **secure rollers** during setting and for **dressing long hair**.

Fine hair pins are mainly used for **dressing hair up** and are available in several shades to **match the client's hair colour**.

Hair grips, like **fine hair pins**, are available in a **variety of colours** and are mostly used for **long hair dressings**.

Setting nets are used to keep rollers and pin curls in place while the client is under the dryer.

Hair nets are often made from real hair and come in a variety of colours and shades. They are very useful for **show** or **photographic** work to keep long hair smooth and in place when dressing into pleats/rolls, etc., as they are extremely fine and barely visible if used correctly.

Styling and finishing products

Setting aids

Setting aids serve two main purposes: to protect the hair from the heat of the hairdryer, and to prevent the hair from absorbing moisture – which will, in turn, prolong the life of the style. They do this by coating the hair with a fine, water-soluble plastic film.

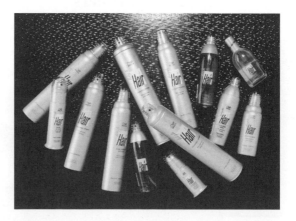

Setting lotions/gel sprays

These come in liquid form and can be runny. Gel sprays are a modern form of setting lotion and usually come in non-aerosol spray bottles. They will give a firm hold and are applied to wet hair before setting.

> **Remember**
>
> Humidity in the atmosphere can cause your hairstyle to drop. The use of styling and finishing products will act as a barrier to moisture in the atmosphere.

Mousse
Also used when wet setting, this gives a softer result than setting lotions.

Gel/sculpting lotions
These have a thicker consistency than lotions. They do not run and are ideal for sculpting or moulding the hair – for example, when creating finger waves.

Thermo-active sprays
These are used when dry-setting with Velcro or heated rollers to help hold the style. They are applied to clean, dry hair either before or after placing rollers, depending on the hair length. When setting longer hair, it is better to apply them before setting to ensure an even curl strength.

Dressing hair

Wax
This gives the strongest hold and is used to prevent static, give definition and mould the hair. It can be quite heavy and can make the hair look lank and greasy if too much is applied.

Frequent use can also cause build-up.

Pomades/dressing creams
These have the same uses as wax but are lighter to use, gentler on the hair and do not leave build-up.

Shine sprays
These will give hair shine and help prevent static. They should be used sparingly as they can make the hair look greasy.

Moisturisers
Products such as Wella System Professional Active Repair fluid, often called **serums**, are moisturising products formulated for use on longer hair to smooth the hair, giving shine and accentuating the style.

Hair sprays
These are used to finish the style and to help control longer hair when dressing up.

> **Remember**
>
> It is important to know how and when to use styling and finishing products.

Setting techniques

Wet setting

Setting the hair when wet will give a firmer, longer-lasting result, which is ideal when creating structured styles such as finger waves or when working on fine hair which does not hold a set well.

Dry setting

This method involves setting clean, dry hair and gives a softer, more casual result, which is ideally suited to today's fashion styles. The two most popular methods are to use **Velcro rollers** or **heated rollers**. Methods of winding are the same as when using conventional setting rollers, with the finished result being determined by the curl direction, volume created and size of rollers used.

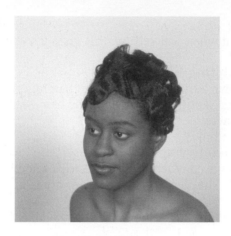

Traditional setting methods

Traditional methods include setting on rollers, pin-curling and finger-waving. These are essential skills, learned during training, which can all be adapted and incorporated into classic, fashion and alternative hair dressings.

Alternative setting methods

Alternative setting methods include spiral winding using Molton Browners, chopsticks or rags. This method of winding is the same as when spiral winding for a perm. (Chapter 3 gives a description of how to carry out the wind.)

Creative styling and finishing

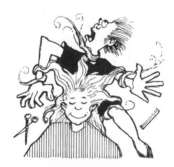

Once the basic skills of setting have been mastered, the techniques can be adapted as desired to create classic, fashion or alternative styles. It is often possible to combine a variety of setting techniques – rollers, pin curls and finger waves – on one head to produce a specific 'look'.

Preparing hair for dressing out

Points to remember when dressing out:

- **Remove any large earrings or necklaces** that the client is wearing, in case they become entangled in the client's long hair.
- If back-combing is required, use only at the **root area** and not through mid-lengths and ends. When dressing the hair down, try to limit back-combing to the **crown area** only.
- If tying hair up in **pony tails**, use covered bands to prevent damage to hair.
- If using ornamentation, make sure it **balances** the style rather than overwhelms it.
- Hairspray – use a fast-drying hairspray with medium hold when working and switch to a stronger hold to finish.

Tip: instead of buying elastic bands, make your own using fine, rolled dressmakers elastic – cut to size and hand knot as required.

Remember

Allow hair to cool completely before dressing out. Taking rollers out when the hair is still warm will loosen the curl, giving a softer result.

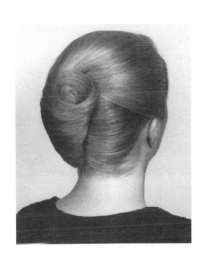

Choosing brushes for dressing out

Smooth styles

Use an open-tufted brush such as isnis or paddle when brushing hair out to remove roller marks. Smooth the hair into position and back-brush the crown area if required.

Curly styles

For a more casual finish, dress out the hair using your fingers or an Afro comb to separate the curls. Remember, brushing can produce a frizzy look. See colour plate 8.

Dressing long hair up

Dressing longer hair up requires more practice but again, once basic styles and techniques of braiding and dressing have been achieved, it is possible to build on them and create many different results, depending on the occasion and client requirements. See colour plate 8.

A pleat

Back-comb or back-brush to create volume at roots (see Figure 1 below). Leaving out the top section, comb one side of the hair smoothly towards the centre back and secure with a line of interlocking grips, finishing just under the crown area (Figure 2). Brush or comb the other side of the hair, then twist or fold the hair under, ensuring that the pleat is in the middle, and secure firmly with grips or pins (Figure 3). Smooth over the top hair, blend it in with the pleated back hair and grip firmly (Figure 4).

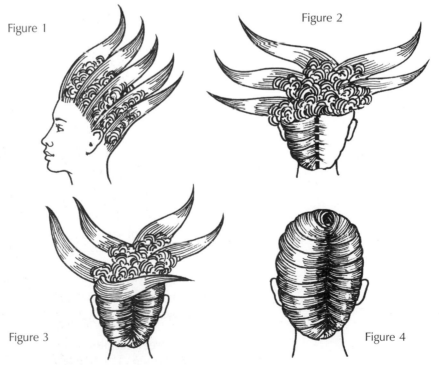

Figure 1

Figure 2

Figure 3

Figure 4

Check the front of the dressing for balance and shape, using the end of a tail comb to lift the hair if necessary. Use finishing spray as desired and check that no pins or grips are visible.

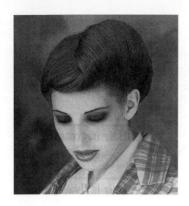

A roll

This is a horizontal roll of hair, which may be worn at the back, sides or on the top of the head.

Begin by back-combing or brushing to create volume (Figure 1). Smooth over the top hair in the direction of the finished dressing to decide on the height of the finished roll. Place a row of interlocking hairgrips firmly along the scalp in a line just under where the roll will be placed (Figure 2).

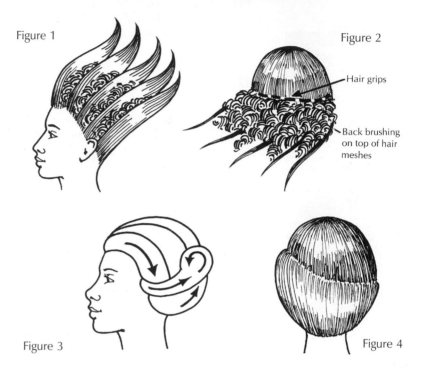

Figure 1

Figure 2

Hair grips

Back brushing on top of hair meshes

Figure 3

Figure 4

Starting at one side of the head, brush or comb the hair up towards the grips and fold the hair over. Tuck it under to form a horizontal roll and grip it firmly as you work from one side to the other. Work around the head, checking in the mirror for shape and balance before you complete the result (Figures 3 and 4).

Simple chignon

Ideal for using on very long, thick, heavy hair.

Pull the hair into a sleek pony tail at the nape of the neck and secure with a band. Tie the hair into a knot but do not pull the ends of the hair through the centre of the knot; this will create the chignon shape. Flick the ends of the hair under the 'knot' and secure with hair grips. Cover the chignon with a fine net and pin/grip into place to finish.

Curly hair – casual updo

For this style you are trying to create a casual soft shape. The 'template' is a triangular shape.

Divide hair into three sections – two front sections from a centre parting, ear to ear across crown. The whole back of the head is the third section.

Twist the back section of the hair into a loose pleat and pin, leaving curls at the crown. Twist the base of small sections of hair sticking out of pleat and grip into place to create an even shape.

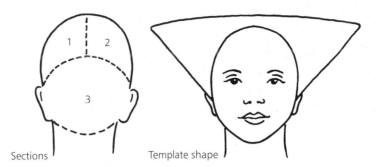

Sections   Template shape

Casual updo

For the side sections use a two-pronged setting pin in a chopstick action, swirl the hair around the ends of the pin, put into place and secure by pushing into the root area to build up the shape. Continue in this manner with all side sections until a good shape has been created. Do not use wax to finish as this can make the hair heavy, causing the style to collapse – use hairspray to give definition to the curls.

Added hair

False hair pieces are ideal for adding bulk and length to hair, whether dressing it up or down. When false hair is used, make sure it is correctly positioned and securely attached. Many hair pieces come with combs or clip attachments for securing in place but hair grips can also be used for added security.

Health and safety when setting and dressing

As with any other hairdressing service there are many health and safety considerations to be aware of. Always follow the basic rules when setting and dressing hair, including:

- Prepare all tools and equipment before use – check manufacturers' instructions if unsure.
- Ensure that you know how to use any electrical equipment, e.g. heated rollers.
- Make a visual check of electrical equipment before using to ensure it is safe to use and minimise the risk of accidents.
- Protect the client and her clothing throughout the service.
- Remember COSHH regulations – store, handle and dispose of all products used according to manufacturers' instructions and salon policy.
- Sterilise all tools and equipment before use to help prevent cross-infection and spreading infections to yourself and others.
- Maintain a professional image by keeping work areas clean and tidy.

HEALTH MATTERS
Always carry out a thorough check for any infections or infestations before commencing. Remember, these are easily spread.

To do

- List the different tools and equipment you may use when dressing hair and the best method of sterilising for each.

Salon professional image

The image of the salon is portrayed through the type and standard of work (or services) it provides to its clients.

Benefits to be gained by enhancing the professional image of the salon include increased salon business, increased client take-up of new and existing salon services, greater client satisfaction and the potential to become involved with new opportunities such as hair shows, seminars, etc.

To do

- Think of some other benefits to be gained by enhancing your salon's image and list some further ways of enhancing the image of your salon.

Test your knowledge

1 Why is it important to consider **hair fall** and **hair growth patterns** when planning a style?
2 List the **health and safety** points to consider with regard to the use of equipment.
3 What are your responsibilities under **COSHH regulations** regarding styling and finishing products?
4 Why should you **check electrical equipment** before using?
5 Why is it important to **avoid cross-infection** and infestation?
6 Give examples of **classic**, **fashion** and **alternative** looks.
7 What are the best **rollers** to use on bleached or highly porous hair?
8 What adverse effect can excessive use of **heated styling equipment** have on the hair?
9 What effect will the **amount of rollers** used have on the finished style?
10 What effect does the **size of rollers** used have on the end result?
11 When would you use **Molton Browners**?
12 Why should you allow the hair to **cool** before dressing out?
13 How can **humidity** affect the finished style?
14 What would be the best brush to use when dressing hair into a **smooth style**?
15 Why should hair sections be **brushed thoroughly** before dressing?
16 When would you use the following products:
   - Gel
   - Wax
   - Dressing cream
   - Moisturisers
   - Shine spray
   - Finishing spray
17 How can you ensure that the client is happy with the end result?
---

10 Promotions and shows

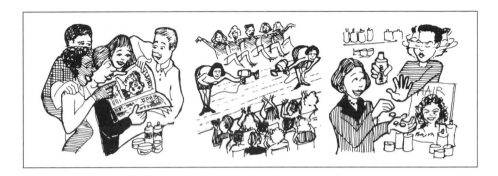

This chapter includes all the required knowledge for Unit 15, which applies to loading the work of teams and individuals to achieve objectives

Setting objectives

In order to increase salon business, it is essential to take an active part in promoting the salon, the staff and the services you offer.

When arranging any type of promotional activity it is important to set out and plan the **objectives** or **outcomes** of the activity. The objectives are to:

- **Plan** the work for your team or individual staff members
- **Assess** the work for your team or individual staff members
- **Give feedback** on the work to all your team members

Why do a promotion?

The main reasons for promoting a salon are:

- To **promote and enhance** the salon image
- To make clients **aware of the services the salon offers**
- To **attract new clients**
- To **encourage existing clients** to return
- To **motivate staff** for personal growth and achievement and become part of a successful team

Discussions with management and colleagues will help identify areas that need development and establish the objectives of your promotional activity.

How can you promote your salon?

There are many ways in which to promote a salon.

Short term
- **Displays**, e.g. retail display in salon
- **Special offers**, such as:
  - free product samples
  - discount prices on services

Medium term
- **Advertising**, e.g.:
  - local newspapers
  - local television/radio
  - leaflet drops
  - within salon, using promotional posters/photographs of work by staff
- **Demonstrations**, e.g. to professional and non-professional groups
- **Shows**, e.g. to small and large groups (Women's Institute, Girl Guides)

To do

- List the ways in which you could best promote your salon, and the main objectives of each method.

Targeting the promotion

The nature of the target group you wish to attract will influence the promotional activity you choose to present.

When planning a promotional activity, consider the following questions:

- Do you want to attract the general public in order to expand your client base? If so, **what age groups** do you want to appeal to – a specific age range, or a wider cross-section of the community?
- Do you want to attract **female clients, male clients, or both?**
- Will your promotion be aimed at **new clients, existing clients or both?**
- What is your **product/service?** Do you have a clear idea of what, or who, you are trying to promote?
- **When will the promotion take place?** Will clients need advance notification, e.g. for a show demonstration?
- **Why should they buy/use the product or service?** What are the benefits to them? (Remember that **listing the benefits** of the product is an important part of selling.)
- **How is it to be used?** In the case of a product or service, clients and customers need information.

Remember

You need to consider your company's
- **organisational objectives** – is it to increase your clientele or to raise the profile of the salon?
- **organisational policies** – are staff expected to work on their day off? Are staff going to be paid overtime?

To do

- Look at the three groups listed below and consider the best forms of promotion to suit the needs of each:
  - Young adults
  - Working mothers
  - Male clients

Important points to remember

To ensure the success of any promotional activity, planning and preparation are vital to gain everyone's support and commitment. It is a good idea to have a **detailed plan** showing what is to be done, by whom and when. It should include:

- **Dates and times** of any team meetings
- **Jobs** to be carried out, and by whom
- **Responsibilities** of those involved – i.e.
  - those with **line responsibility** – who have to plan and report back to their line manager
  - those with **functional responsibility** – who have specific functions within various areas of work and may not be part of the line management e.g. a part-time specialist media consultant
- **Rehearsal** dates (if required)
- **Deadline** dates

It could also include information on available resources and budget details. Remember to update your plan on a regular basis, making a note of any changes.

A sample plan for a hair and beauty show is shown on page 160.

Motivating staff

Involving members of staff in putting together and presenting any form of promotional activity is a good way to motivate them.

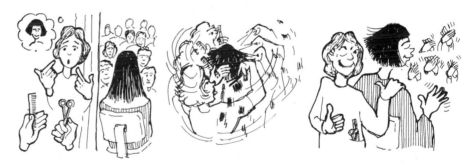

The following are proven motivators:

- Being given **responsibility** with an element of independence
- Being given work that is **creative** and **challenging**
- Having scope for **personal growth** and **achievement**
- Being part of a **successful team**

If staff are motivated, they are more likely to **work hard**, and if they are given specific roles to carry out during the promotional activity, this will help ensure its success and give those involved a **sense of achievement**.

Resources

The next step is to consider the **resources** you will need in order to carry out your promotion successfully. These usually fall into three categories.

- Staffing
- Tools and equipment
- Promotional materials and products

Uxbridge College Hair and Beauty Show

Venue	Hayes site
Date	Sunday April 27th 1999
Time	Doors open 7.00 pm
Seating capacity	200/250

Student responsibilities

Beauty therapy students	Make-up
FT 1st Year Hairdressers	Assisting
FT 2nd Year Hairdressers	Preparation of models
P/T Level III Hairdressers	Organising models/clothes/accessories/preparing models

Staff responsibilities

Line responsibility
Claire Jones — Co-ordinating Beauty Therapy students

Kirsten Harjette — Co-ordinating 2nd Year students, liaising with Marketing, Lighting and Sound

Co-ordination functional responsibility
Stephanie Henderson — Liaising with sponsors and photographers

Show structure

Four main sections:

7.30 pm	Start: 20-minute Introduction
	Scene 1: Black-Sleek lines
	Scene 2: White

Break for refreshments 30 minutes

8.20 pm	Level III: Historical/High Fashion and Fantasy
8.35 pm	Scene 3: Black and White
	Scene 4: Colour and Finale

Staffing

When delegating tasks, always consider the **strengths of the individual(s)**. Remember that you are also giving each individual **authority** and it is important that everyone involved is aware of the **limits of their authority**, what their **responsibilities** are and **when they will be needed**.

To do

- Using your chosen promotional activity, list the various jobs which need doing.
- Match your staff/colleagues to each role.

Tools and equipment

The tools and equipment required will be dependent on the type of promotional activity you have chosen. Advertising through leaflet drops, newspapers, local radio, etc., will need little, if any, equipment, whereas salon displays, demonstrations and shows will require access to specific hairdressing tools and equipment. Always ensure that any tools, equipment, products – and staff – are available not only on the night of the demonstration or show but also during any rehearsals.

Promotional materials and products

Promotional materials include **posters, leaflets, tickets, programmes and vouchers**. These will all have to be printed, and some will be needed sooner than others, so it is a good idea to make up a production schedule for each item, and to give a member of the team responsibility for ensuring that dates are adhered to.

Remember

Make up a list of all the resources you are likely to need throughout the activity.

To celebrate the opening of our new Hairdressing & Beauty Salon,

join us for an evening of Creativity and Innovation with

PATRICK CAMERON

On Tuesday 26th October 1999

at 6.30pm for 7.00pm

RSVP Stephanie Henderson 0181 756 0414

by 7th October

Hayes Centre, Coldharbour Lane, Hayes, Middlesex UB3 3BB

THIS TICKET ADMITS ONE PERSON

Invitation to a salon promotion

If you are promoting a particular product or range of products, make sure that you have **sufficient supplies** in stock for retail, and also for use in demonstrations or shows (including rehearsals). Contact product manufacturers to see if they are willing to provide **free samples** for clients to try, or for use during a demonstration or show.

HEALTH MATTERS

Always take into account health and safety considerations and any other legal requirements when planning your promotional activity. Remember to give a member of the team responsibility for overseeing health and safety.

| To do |

■ Re-read Chapter 6, which deals with government laws and acts relating to hairdressing, and write a list of the ones that may influence your promotion.

Demonstrations and shows

Two major factors when deciding on the format of a demonstration or hair show are the type and size of audience you wish to attract.

Demonstrations

Demonstrations are usually aimed at smaller groups. Audiences will fall into two categories: **professional** and **non-professional**.

Professional groups
These could be made up of your staff or hairdressers from other salons – either experienced stylists or trainees. For groups of this type, the content of the demonstration would be more **technical** – perhaps a demonstration of a particular technique or skill.

Remember to take into account the abilities of the group when planning the content of the demonstration.

Non-professional groups
Non-professional audiences can be from specific organisations such as Women's Institutes, Girl Guides or mother-and-toddler groups. The age of the audience needs to be considered when planning this type of event.

These demonstrations would be more **informal** and could include hair and beauty make-overs, question-and-answer sessions on hair and beauty, one-to-one consultations, and also information on the services your salon offers.

Although the two groups are very different, the methods of **preparation** and **presentation** of the demonstration are similar. See Chapter 11 for information on how to plan and present a demonstration to a small group.

Shows

If you choose to present a larger show it is important to reach a **good cross-section** of the community. One possibility would be to involve a local charity and use the show as a fund-raising event.

The size of the presentation will also influence your choice of venue, the content of the show and the price of entry tickets.

Content
One of the first decisions that must be made is the **format** and **content** of the show. A **brainstorming session** with members of your team is a good way of coming up with ideas.

Some possibilities include:

- Hair and fashion, using mature and young models
- A children's event
- Weddings
- Sports
- Avant-garde
- High fashion
- Historical themes
- Make-over spot

To do

- Think of some other 'themes' that could be incorporated into your show.

Once you have decided on the content of the show, your next step is to plan the sequence and pace of the delivery. In discussion with members of your team, decide on the sequence of the themes chosen and the length of time each segment should last.

Remember, you are **showing your skills to prospective clients**. Don't rush the delivery or it will be difficult for the audience to take in what they are seeing. On the other hand, don't let things drag on for too long or the audience may lose interest.

Rehearsals will give a good idea as to how things are progressing and allow adjustments to be made.

Putting a show together

There will be various costs involved in putting a hair show together and these will depend greatly on the size of the presentation planned.

Costs may include:

- Cost of hiring the venue
- Printing of promotional materials
- Publicity – advertisements in local newspapers, etc.
- Accessories – hair ornamentation, hairpieces, jewellery, etc.
- Hair products – shampoos, styling products, etc.
- Sundry items – dry-cleaning, laundry, refreshments, etc.
- Fees for helpers

One way of reducing costs would be to **involve local businesses** in the event. For example:

- Local **clothes/shoe stores** could be asked to loan outfits
- **Design students** from the local college might help with designing **promotional materials**; fashion students could design outfits for avant-garde themes
- **Bridal shops** could lend outfits for a wedding theme
- **Record stores** may help with music
- **Local radio** may give free advertising

Example of Cost Estimates for a College Hair Show

Lighting and sound £150

Hair accessories £80

Video production £40

Photography £50

Programmes . . . . Donated by Wella

Security . . . . All staff gave services free

Refreshments £150

Hall hire . . . . Free

Hair sundries (gel, spray, etc.) £20

Flowers £30

Raffle prize . . . . CD player from Wella was on bonus offer

Printing costs £20

- **Local papers** may print an article about the salon and the show
- Inviting local businesses and hair product manufacturers/retailers to advertise in the programme will help **reduce printing costs**
- If you don't know any make-up artists, get in touch with **local beauty salons or freelance artists**

Choosing the date

The timing of the show may be influenced by several factors:

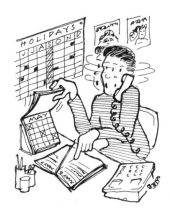

- **Availability of the venue.** You may be restricted by available dates so check with the venue before setting a firm date.
- **Holidays.** Remember to take into account staff, school and public holidays.
- **Time of year.** If planning a show during the winter months, remember that the weather may affect the size of the audience.

Choosing the venue

Several factors will need to be considered when choosing a suitable venue:

- It must be **easily accessible**. Are there **good public transport** and **car parking** facilities? Facilities and access for the **disabled**?
- Is the hall **big enough** for your needs? Remember to find out the **maximum audience capacity**.
- Does it have the **facilities** you require? These will include a **stage area,**

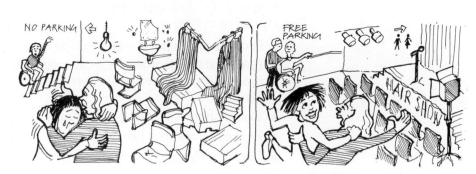

adequate seating, a **changing area** with room for preparation of models, suitable **water** and **power** supply and **appropriate lighting**. Remember to check out the **sound system**. Is there one you can use, or will you have to supply your own?

- How much will it **cost**? Are there **reduced rates** for certain days of the week or times of the year? If possible, check out several places – sports centres, community centres, school halls or hotels – and **compare prices** before deciding on a venue.
- Are you allowed to use the venue for **rehearsals**?
- Will the venue be **ready for use** on the date required (for example, will seating be provided), or are you responsible for setting up?

Publicising the show

There are many ways to publicise the show and it is important that whichever methods you choose will reach a large number of people. Possible ideas include **mailshots** to homes within the area, or **leaflets/fliers** delivered with local free papers. A **press release** or **advertisement** in the local papers with details of date and time will create interest, as would a spot on a **local radio** show. **Promotional posters** displayed throughout the area are also a good idea.

To do

- Think of some good places to display promotional posters.

Allocating jobs

Listed below are some of the roles which need to be undertaken by members of your team:

- **Show co-ordinator**. This involves overseeing the whole event and liaising with all those involved in the show.
- **Compere** – needs to be comfortable speaking to a large group of people and a good communicator.
- **Stylists** – must be confident working in front of people, competent and able to choose styles for models that can be easily converted backstage. They also need to be able to work quickly – time is often limited.
- **Juniors** – needed to assist backstage with minor tasks and preparation work. Must be able to take instruction, work with minimum support and use initiative.
- **Make-up artists** – needed to make up models. (*Note:* If any make-up artists are new to you, make sure you see examples of their work before agreeing to use them. Try approaching local colleges/beauty salons for help.)
- **Dresser** – needed to co-ordinate outfits and accessories.
- **Models** – must be confident and able to perform routines and walk catwalk without embarrassment.
- **Choreographer** – needed to plan routines, timing of models, etc.
- **Music co-ordinator** – needs to be familiar with music systems and able to suggest suitable music for each theme.

To do

- Using the list of roles above, consider the tasks each person would be expected to carry out before and during the show.

Problems

As with any activity, problems may arise. Below are some problems which may arise and how to avoid them.

Troubleshooting

Problem	Solution
Jobs not carried out to schedule.	Allocate jobs to specific members of staff with deadline dates for completion.
Promotional materials not ready on time.	Make sure printers/manufacturers know when materials are required.
Resources, e.g. stock, not available.	Ensure extra stock, accessories and equipment are ordered prior to promotion date.
Models let you down.	Have standby models available.
Staff/models late for rehearsals.	Give everyone involved a printed list of dates, times and places of rehearsals.

To do

■ Think of ways in which to resolve the problems below, and think of some other problems which may arise and how to solve them.
 – You've run out of promotional materials and products
 – The venue has been double-booked

Evaluation and assessment of the activity

Evaluation and assessment of your promotional activity will help you to gauge its success and learn lessons for future promotions.

Reasons for evaluation and assessment

- **Qualitative.** To gain feedback on the activity. Was the quality of the promotion better than previous promotions? As good as, or worse than, those of your competitors?
- **Quantitative.** To judge the effect on salon training. Were the resources – tools, equipment, products and promotional materials – adequate?

There are many methods of evaluation. Some examples are given below:

- **Feedback/discussion sessions** with other members of the team
- **Informal talks with clients** – these will give a general overview of how people felt about the promotion
- Keeping **a record of new clients** visiting the salon
- **Monitoring sales of services or products promoted** to see if there is an increase in demand
- **Questionnaires** – these give more structured feedback and can be designed for both staff and clients to complete

Managers need to keep records of evaluations and assessments to be able to justify and improve future promotions.

Whatever form of evaluation you choose, the following topics should be included:

- Did the activity achieve its aims and objectives? (Was it **valid**?)
- Costs involved: how was money spent? Could it have been better spent elsewhere?
- What you think worked well? (Were the techniques **current**?)
- Areas that could be improved? (Was it **authentic**?)
- Content: would you use the same format again?
- Was there anything that should be added, or left out, next time? (Was it **sufficient**?)

If a hair show/demonstration:

- Was the pace too fast/slow/OK?
- Method of delivery: was it clear and concise? Did the audience understand what was going on?

On page 170 you will find an example of an evaluation questionnaire.

To do

■ Once you have chosen your promotional activity, design an evaluation questionnaire which could be given to clients and/or staff to complete.

Reviewing the evaluation questionnaire

The completed evaluation questionnaire sheets need to be compiled by adding up the amounts of 'yes' and 'no' responses to give percentages. For example:

> **Q1** Did you enjoy the show?

If 80 people attended and 75 answered 'yes' and 5 answered 'no' then 94% enjoyed the show but 6% did not.

Audience comments should also be clearly and logically listed, e.g. it needs to be stated only once that five people said that the commentary could have been a little louder.

Both **positive** and **negative** feedback of a general nature can be given through:

- **General discussion – informally** in the staff rest room during breaks or **formally** during staff meetings.
- **In a written form** –through **staff appraisals** (see Chapter 14), where confidentiality is needed (especially if feedback is negative). Always make your feedback constructive and put the other person at ease – most people realise when they have made a mistake and are only too anxious to improve any future performances. Allow the staff to provide their own suggestions on how they could improve and list the ideas as part of their future goals.

Hair and Beauty Show Evaluation*

Please spare two minutes to complete this questionnaire to let us know how you felt about the show. Please tick the Yes or No boxes:

		Yes	*No*
1	Did you enjoy the show?	☐	☐
2	Could you see everything clearly?	☐	☐
3	Could you hear everything that was said?	☐	☐
4	Did you find it easy to purchase the tickets?	☐	☐
5	Was the Level 2 (the full-time students') work up to the standard you expected?	☐	☐
6	Was the Level 3 (mature students') work up to the standard you expected?	☐	☐
7	Did you find the college map helpful?	☐	☐
8	Was the price of the ticket good value for money?	☐	☐
9	Were the refreshments sufficient?	☐	☐
10	If we put on another show next year, will you come again?	☐	☐

Please feel free to add any other comments below:

_____

_____

_____

Name _____

Signature _____ Date _____

* A photocopiable version of this form appears on page 245.

Test your knowledge

1 List the main **reasons for promoting a salon**.
2 List the **ways of promoting a salon**.
3 How do you decide on what type of **promotional activity to use**?
4 Describe the difference between someone who works within the **line manager's responsibility** and someone who has a **functional responsibility**, and the **implications** these differences may have **for planning the work**.
5 Why is it important to **plan and prepare** a promotional activity?
6 Why is it important to **involve staff/colleagues**?
7 How would you **suit staff to specific tasks**?
8 List the ways of **publicising** your promotion.
9 Why is it a **good idea to evaluate** promotions and shows?
10 How can you evaluate the success of your promotion to ensure that it is a **fair and objective assessment**?
11 How could both **negative** and **positive feedback** be given and why is it important?
12 Which type of feedback should always be **confidential** and why?
13 How does the evaluation of your promotion **apply to you** (the manager)?

11 Demonstrating and instructing

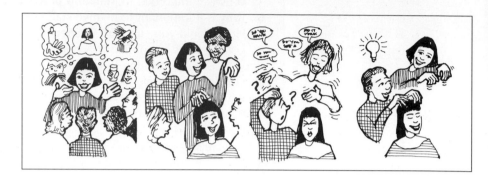

The importance of preparation

In order to demonstrate to or instruct learners in hairdressing techniques, it is essential to prepare thoroughly. This includes not only all the practical aspects of making sure students can see clearly and that all your tools and equipment are accessible but also considering your **attitude** towards your learners.

Learners must feel **safe** in their environment. This means that you need to support, guide and encourage them at every stage. Never brush aside their offerings or belittle their work as being out of date or of little value. Always stress the positive side of any previous learning experience. For example, someone will always say, 'That's not the way my salon does it'. A good reply would be: 'That's interesting, but I am going to show you another way of achieving the same result.'

Demonstrating (showing techniques and skills)

In order to demonstrate a skill, you first need to analyse it by breaking it down into **small parts** and **listing the sequence** in which it has to be learned.

The demonstration needs to accurately reflect **real practice** and to maximise learning. For example, it would be a waste of time to expect someone to watch a 1½-hour spiral perm being wound from start to finish without other learning activities going on at the same time.

Demonstrations need to be as realistic as possible, with **any differences between the demonstration and real-life practice highlighted**. For example, you should slow down your massage techniques when shampooing to clearly show how your fingers are moving.

A demonstration shampoo

Below is a breakdown of the tasks you will need to cover in your demonstration:

- Prepare all tools and equipment needed
- Gown up the client comfortably
- Disentangle the hair
- Analyse the hair and scalp
- Consult with the client and choose a shampoo
- Check the water supply
- Check that the temperature of the water is suitable for the client, then wet the hair thoroughly
- Apply the shampoo using the correct movements
- Massage the hair and scalp using the correct movements, repeating if necessary
- Rinse the hair thoroughly
- Apply a surface conditioner if necessary; disentangle and rinse the hair if needed
- Remove any excess water from the hair
- Bring the client to an upright position so that they are dry and comfortable

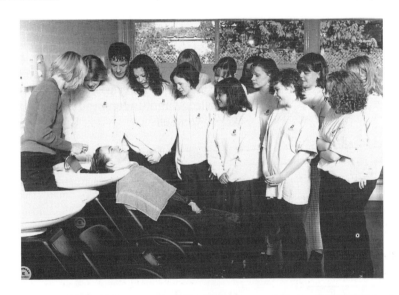

A demonstration of shampooing techniques

Make sure that the learners are comfortable about asking questions and make appropriate comments during the demonstration, e.g. 'This is the shampoo I have chosen for this client. What type of shampoo would you choose in your salon on this occasion?'

Give the learners the opportunity to **practise the skill** soon after the demonstration. For example, they will often need a further demonstration of the massage techniques before they can apply the correct pressure.

Always choose the site and location of the demonstration to allow **optimum visibility**. Make sure the learners are close enough, or arrange any moveable dressing table mirrors strategically for good vision.

Remember to **minimise distractions** (e.g. turn the radio off) and interruptions (e.g. tell the other staff to interrupt only if there is an emergency).

Demonstrating to individuals and groups

Learners often feel more threatened in a one-to-one situation than in a group, so if you are demonstrating to an individual you will need to spend time putting them at their ease. For a small-to-medium-size group of 4–10 people, either arrange seats beforehand for optimum visibility or ask the group to stand where they can see all aspects of the demonstration clearly.

To do

- Write up a 'step by step' demonstration for:
  - A set
  - A perm or relaxer
  - A colour technique, e.g. regrowth or foils
  - A basic haircut
  - A long hair dressing
  - A blow dry

Remember to include an explanation of your choice of equipment and notes on the location used.

Questioning techniques

Always prepare any questions – and the answers to them – beforehand. Consider what the learners **must know** about the topic (like the essential knowledge and understanding requirements of NVQ), rather than what you know yourself.

Written and oral questions

Questions can be asked in **written form**, with the learners writing down their answers, or they can be **oral questions** which are asked by you and answered verbally by the learners.

Whichever method you choose, make sure that the questions are unambiguous and use straightforward language. It is better to ask short, snappy questions than lengthy ones covering several different aspects.

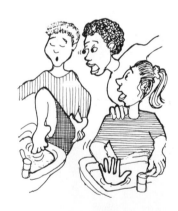

Remember

Questions that are asked orally can be highly stressful for learners.

Open and closed questions

Try to use **open** rather than closed questions. For example, an open question could be: 'Why did I check the water temperature on the inside of my wrist?' Answer – 'It is a more sensitive area of the skin to judge the heat of the water'.

A closed question would be: 'Did I remember to check the water temperature on the inside of my wrist?' Answer – 'Yes' (or 'No'), which does not check understanding.

Learners can be confused or demoralised by what they perceive to be aggressive or unfair questioning. Always make sure you give them the information they need to know either before or during the demonstration before asking any questions.

There are different styles of questions:

- They may be **factual** – e.g. 'What shampoo should be used for dry hair?'
- They may concern **reasons for a certain action or decision** – e.g. 'Why did I choose a surface conditioner as well as a shampoo for this client with dry, long hair?'
- They may concern things that **might happen** – e.g. 'If I was going to perm today, what type of shampoo would I choose for this client with long, dry hair?'
- They may be **follow-up questions**, to check the learners' understanding of an earlier question – e.g. 'Well, let me put it another way. What shampoo out of the range I showed you today should be used for dry hair?'

Keep your questions simple and easy to understand. Speak slowly and clearly with a friendly, helpful tone.

To do

- Make up a list of six questions and answers related to your demonstration. Try them out on a colleague before doing your demonstration.
- Re-read Chapter 6 regarding the laws that affect you at work.

Health and safety

Before and during a demonstration always consider health, safety and good practice. Here is a general checklist.

Hygiene and infections
Check the client's hair and scalp for infections. Use only clean and sterile tools, equipment and materials.

Sharps
Keep scissors and razor blades closed and in a safe place when not in use.

Water and electricity
Check all electrical appliances for safety and correct insulation. Do not use electrical appliances near water.

Trailing leads
Ensure that no-one – you, your client or the learners – could trip over trailing electrical leads on the salon floor.

Spillages
Mop up all spillages immediately to prevent falls.

Personal and client protection
Make sure the client is gowned up adequately and that you are wearing the correct protective equipment, e.g. gloves and/or aprons.

First aid
Make sure you know where the first aid box is located and who is responsible for first aid in the salon.

COSHH
Read up the rules concerning the storage and use of hazardous chemicals in the salon – e.g. on mixing chemicals in a ventilated area.

Egress
Always remind learners how to find the fire exits, and make sure that no obstacles such as boxes or bags could hinder a fast exit in the event of an emergency.

Instructing ('talking through' techniques and skills)

You need to accurately identify what it is that learners **need to know and do**.

For example, to shampoo to a professional standard, they should be able to:

- Prepare and gown up the client correctly.
- Select the products, tools and scalp massage techniques based on the client consultation.
- Ensure that the water temperature and flow are comfortable for the client and suited to the needs of the hair and scalp.
- Shampoo correctly and repeat if required.
- Make sure that the head and scalp are left clean and free from shampoo and excess moisture.
- Use surface conditioners only if needed, and apply and remove them appropriately.
- Complete by leaving the hair tangle-free and undamaged.

You also need to accurately identify your **learning outcomes**, e.g.:

- Do you want your learners to be able to shampoo to a commercial standard, but still ask for guidance on the product choice?
- Do you want your learners to shampoo to an NVQ Level 2 standard with a thorough background knowledge of product ranges and use, and the technical pH values of products?

> **Remember**
>
> Always put your learners at ease. Remember to smile at them occasionally, and praise their correct answers or actions.
> Nothing succeeds like success!

To instruct learners appropriately, you have to know what level they have already reached in their training. For example, a new Saturday girl in a salon who has never observed professional shampooing needs very clear step-by-step instruction, whereas a group of experienced shampooists may need only certain points highlighted to reinforce their knowledge before being taken a stage further.

You also need to check your learners' understanding regularly and modify your instruction accordingly. For example:

- The new Saturday girl may require two different shampoo demonstrations, the first on short, fine, curly hair, the second on long, thick, straight hair.
- The experienced shampooists may need only confirmation of their techniques, but further clarification of all the products available.

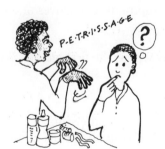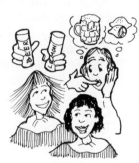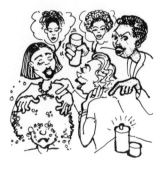

All learners require **timely feedback**. This needs to be given in a **positive and encouraging manner** to show them how they are progressing towards their learning outcomes.

Feedback can be given **orally** or by marking **written questions or assignments**. If learners have not yet achieved their goals, always explain why, and how they can proceed to become competent.

Troubleshooting

If your feedback shows that learners have not grasped the key points of your instruction, the reasons could be as follows:

- Your delivery was too hurried, unclear or too much information was given.
- You did not analyse your learners' capabilities properly or pitched your instruction either too high or too low.
- There was too much background noise, or you were constantly interrupted during your instruction.
- The learners had language problems – maybe English is their second language, or they have dyslexia and problems with written instructions.

These factors need to be explored and rectified, and your instruction altered accordingly. For example:

- **Don't** get impatient when learners are slow to grasp the point.
- **Do** explain things carefully, moving from the **known** to the **unknown**.
- Teach small areas in **logical sequence**, adding each new piece of information to the last piece.
- **Don't use jargon** – e.g. words like 'effleurage' – unless appropriate. If you must use technical terms, write them on a flipchart or give a handout to explain what they mean.

Just as a demonstration technique needs to be sequenced, so an **instruction technique** needs to be clearly **summarised**.

To do

- Write up the range of instructions needed for a blow dry.
- State your learner's learning outcomes.
- Describe how you would check their understanding and progress.

Supplementary information in the form of handouts, **visual aids** such as OHPs and transparencies (for note-taking), quizzes, worksheets or highlighting important points in a textbook (such as *Basic Hairdressing* by Stephanie Henderson) will help to reinforce key learning points.

Checking understanding

You can check your learners' understanding and progress in the following ways:

- By **observing** them perform the task and **recording** your comments
- By observing the products of their performance such as **client record cards** or **completed consultation sheets**

Remember

Learning should always be a positive and enjoyable experience.

- By **orally asking questions**
- By giving **written questions**
- By setting small **projects, assignments or case studies** using hypothetical examples

Instructing individuals and groups

Remember to spend more time relaxing an individual learner. A small group of 4–10 will feel less threatened. You do not have to give direct instruction to groups. By giving sub-groups of 2–3 people a small problem-solving task, and asking a spokesman from each sub-group to report back, communication barriers can be broken down.

For example, having described a set of hair-care products, you might ask each sub-group of 2–3 people to discuss and write down which types of shampoo and surface conditioner would be suitable for normal, dry, greasy and dandruff-affected hair. Give them 10 minutes to complete the task and then comment on their answers, perhaps by listing them on a flipchart to reinforce the correct responses.

Test your knowledge

1. What is the difference between **demonstrating** and **instructing** techniques?
2. Give two ways in which you could **put your learners at ease** during a teaching session.
3. Why is it important to use **appropriate language** for different learners?
4. Why is it important to **prepare** your demonstration in a **step-by-step** manner?
5. Describe the different styles of **oral questions** that may be used during a demonstration.
6. Give nine examples of how **Health and Safety legislation** and **good practice** need to be considered during teaching.
7. When you are instructing learners, how do you decide what the **learner's needs** will be?
8. Give two examples of different **learning outcomes** from the same instructed topic.
9. Why is it important to give **constructive feedback**?
10. Describe two examples of factors that could **inhibit learning** and how you could overcome them.
11. List five methods you could use to **check** your **learners' understanding and progress**.

12 Assessing performance (D32)

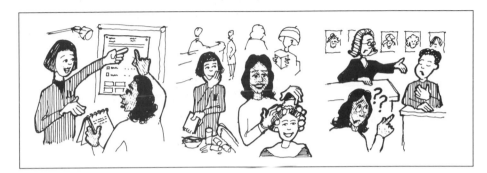

The assessor's role

This chapter is about assessing a candidate's performance (i.e. their practical work, including some records). Chapter 13 is about assessing candidates using differing sources of evidence (i.e. records of their work which may not necessarily be seen when you assess them, such as projects or written questions).

Once you have been assessed and provided all the required evidence for Level 3, Units 12 and 13 (the additional units), you will be a **qualified D32/D33 assessor**. This is often part of a supervisor's role, but **you must hold this certificate** in order for your assessments to be accepted by your approved NVQ assessment centre.

In order to assess a candidate, you must:

1 Select a candidate and choose what is to be assessed
2 Agree an assessment plan with the candidate
3 Observe the candidate doing the work
4 Gather evidence and question the candidate on it
5 Judge the evidence and make your assessment decision
6 Give your candidate feedback and record it

Who's who in the assessment process

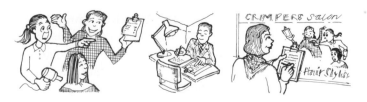

Roles and responsibilities

1. The candidate – i.e. the trainee (registered on an NVQ course) seeking accreditation

It is the responsibility of the **candidate** undertaking the award to ensure that he/she is able to:

- **Identify units, elements and performance criteria** that are to be **assessed** and **possible sources of evidence**.
- **Perform to national standards** in order to be awarded an NVQ.
- **Produce evidence of prior achievement** and current competence.
- Produce the evidence in a **structured format**.

2. The assessor (you)

The assessor must be registered and working towards or hold the D32 and/or D33 certificate.

It is the responsibility of the assessor to:

- **Agree** with the candidate the **evidence presented of prior achievement**.
- Agree an **assessment plan** with the candidate.
- **Brief** the candidate **fully** on the assessment process and ensure that assessments are **fair and reliable**. Explain that internal and external verifiers check all the practical and diverse evidence (oral questions, written questions and projects) at regular intervals to ensure that the candidate is competent in all areas of work.
- **Judge** the candidate's evidence against the national standards and decide whether the candidate has demonstrated **competence**.
- Ensure that the **assessment guidance** given by the awarding body, such as City & Guilds/HTB, and the centre is followed.
- Ensure that all **questions and responses** which are used for the purposes of meeting the evidence requirements and range of standards are recorded.
- Give the candidate **prompt, accurate and constructive feedback**.
- Give the candidate **completed documentation** confirming that she/he has demonstrated competence, if appropriate.
- Give the candidate **constructive feedback** and agree a **new assessment plan** with them if further evidence is required.

3. The internal verifier

The internal verifier is appointed by an approved centre to ensure consistency and quality of assessments within the centre and must hold the D34 certificate.

It is the responsibility of the internal verifier to ensure that:

- All assessors follow the **assessment guidance** given by the City & Guilds/HTB.
- Candidate assessments are sampled to ensure **consistency of assessment**.
- Assessors are given **prompt, accurate and constructive feedback** on their assessment decisions.
- All assessors work to the **same standard** and are **consistent** in their interpretation of national standards and provide them with support and guidance.

- The candidates' **achievement records** and all **centre documentation** meet the standards required by the awarding body.
- Ensure that requests for certificates to the **awarding body** are based on assessments of consistent quality.
- Any **unclear areas of assessment**, such as candidates with special assessment needs, are **referred directly to the external verifier**.

4. External verifiers

These are appointed by awarding bodies – such as City & Guilds/HTB to monitor the work of approved centres and link between the awarding bodies and the centre. They hold the D35 certificate.

It is the responsibility of the external verifier to ensure that :

- **Decisions** on competence are **consistent** across centres.
- The quality of assessments and verification meets the national standards. These are drawn up and agreed by the QCA (Qualifications and Curriculum Authority), and are specified in the Candidate Log Books, the Assessor's Guides and the Assessment of Essential Knowledge and Understanding booklets at Levels 1, 2 and 3.
- Candidate assessments are sampled and assessment and **verification practice is monitored** in centres.
- Regular visits are made to **approved assessment centres**.
- Feedback is given to centres through a **written report**.

1. Select a candidate and what is to be assessed

Remember

There are specified contingency PCs (performance criteria) such as certain hair and scalp abnormalities which need to be assessed.
If these are not available as naturally occurring evidence, then written evidence may be supplemented.

The first step is to **choose a candidate**, i.e. a trainee, who is registered on an NVQ course and who is ready to be assessed – i.e. has been trained and has practised the required skills. Next, select the **elements of competence**, e.g. NVQ Level 2 Hairdressing, 202.1, 202.2, 202.3 Shampoo and Conditioning; 208.1 Working as Part of a Team.

Now carefully read through the nationally specified criteria with the candidate:

- The **performance criteria** (PCs) give a detailed analysis of how the task is done, e.g.:
  2.2 Conditioning:
  – Prepare the client
  – Select the correct products, tools and equipment
  – Apply massage and remove the treatment
  – Leave the hair tangle-free
  – Complete the record card
- The **range statements** describe the different sorts of things that have to be done, e.g.:
  – Surface conditioner
  – Penetrating conditioner
  – Treatment conditioner
  – Include effleurage and petrissage massage
- The **knowledge evidence** describes what the candidate has to know in order to do the work to a competent standard, e.g.:
  – Conditioning products, tools and equipment needed for dry hair, greasy hair and dandruff, and for other salon services such as

protective conditioners used before perming, or corrective conditioners used after perming
- Which hair thickness and lengths of hair need effleurage and which need petrissage massage movements
- How the pH of conditioning products effects hair conditions and further services carried out in the salon
- The effects of water temperature on the hair and scalp

Point out exactly how many observations are needed (listed in the Standards) and identify if all the PCs can be covered, how many of the ranges can be assessed, and if any oral questions will be asked.

It is important to make accurate judgements against **all the criteria** in an element because the candidate will not have completed an element until **all** the PCs, ranges and knowledge evidence have been assessed.

Remember

Make sure that your candidate has a copy of the appeals procedure before you start the assessment.

Equal opportunities

City & Guilds/HTB are two of the **awarding bodies** (i.e. they award the certificates). They also publish **Equal Opportunities Policy Statements**. In practice this means that they are committed to equality of opportunity in education, training and employment. This policy applies to everyone, regardless of gender, age, racial origin, nationality, creed, sexual orientation, marital status, employment status or any disability.

As a qualified assessor, you will need to support this policy by promoting equality of opportunity and avoiding all forms of unfair discrimination.

To do

■ Find out how your assessment centre applies its equal opportunities policies.

Special assessment needs

Remember

When dealing with special assessment needs, always ask the internal verifier for advice.

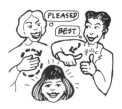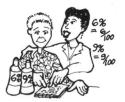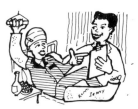

Again, the awarding bodies have policy documents relating to special assessment needs. Here are some examples :

- **Hearing impairment.** The HTB has produced a document relating to the assessment of deaf candidates undertaking reception units. At present it is acceptable for deaf candidates to demonstrate competence through the use of a text phone or telephone relay service, e.g. Typetalk. Other technologies will be reviewed as they are developed
- **Visual and physical impairment**
- **Learning difficulties and medical conditions**
- **Hospitalisation or confinement to home**

2. Agree an assessment plan with the candidate

This plan is drawn up in **agreement with your candidate** and covers at least three elements within one or more units. An example assessment plan is shown on page 184.

To involve your candidate in the assessment process, encourage them to ask questions and seek advice. Use open-ended questions such as 'Which part of the assessment do you find easiest?' Sometimes you will have a candidate who has no experience of presenting evidence for an assessment. You will therefore need to explain the assessment process and the different forms of acceptable evidence. These include:

- **Observation record sheets.**
- **Observation of products** – e.g. client record cards, client consultation sheets (this does not mean *hairdressing* products such as shampoos).
- **Simulation/role-play.** Advice must be sought from the internal and external verifiers regarding the validity and administration of simulations **before** agreeing the assessment plan. If – say – the candidate was not allowed access to the cash till whilst assessing reception, simulation may be acceptable. Using a long-haired tuition head for long hair assessments is not acceptable.
- **Projects/assignments/case studies.**
- **Oral/written questions.** Pre-set written questions must be administered according to the awarding body's regulations (see the booklet *Assessment of Essential Knowledge and Understanding* at your centre).
- **Witness testimonies.**
- **Assessment of prior achievements,** e.g. manufacturers' diplomas. These must be up-to-date and cover the relevant performance criteria and range statements.

You will need to select **appropriate, efficient** methods – for example, observation of the candidate doing the work (naturally occurring evidence) is often quicker and easier (see example assessment plan) than trying to prove that all the range statements have been covered from assessment of prior achievements (e.g. manufacturers' diplomas).

It will help if you can show the candidate completed examples of evidence. Awarding bodies have such examples at the beginning of their candidate log books.

3. Observe the candidate doing the work (i.e. naturally occurring evidence)

Whilst the candidate is working you can **judge** their evidence against the written **performance criteria**. It is important to identify this naturally occurring evidence because assessments must be from **real work activities undertaken by the candidate**. You then need to decide which part of the assessment plan you are going to assess.

To make sure that assessment is appropriate to your candidate's needs, check that:

Example Assessment Plan*

Candidate name	*Karen Overy*
Assessor	*S. Henderson*
Unit no. and title	*202. Shampoo and Condition hair and scalp*
Element no. and title	*202.1, 202.2, 202.3 Work safely and shampoo and surface condition hair and scalp*
Approximate timing of assessment	*30 mins + feedback*

Evidence to be presented:

Natural performance in the workplace i.e. observation	✓	Records of prior achievement	☐
Responses to oral questions	✓	Reports from supervisors in workplaces i.e. witness testimonies	✓
Written projects and assignments	☐		
Review of written records (product evidence) e.g. client record cards	☐	Simulated work activities	☐
Completed written assessment question papers	☐		

Details: *1. Natural performance in the workplace*
Covering performance criteria and 80% of range statements

2. Responses to oral questions
● Covering manufacturer's instructions and range of available shampoos and surface conditioners. Relating them to hair and scalp conditions and other salon services.
● Covering safety aspects e.g. water temperature, working cleanly, avoiding infections and infestations, sterilisation, using electrical

equipment and relating products to COSHH
● Massage techniques related to hair of differing densities and length. How the pH of products affects hair condition and subsequent services.
● Effects of water temperature on the hair and scalp. Effects of using the wrong shampoo and when to repeat the shampoo process.

4. Reports from supervisors in workplaces
Complete two assessments (unobserved by assessor) with witness testimonies signed by supervisor and clients

People involved in my assessment:

Assessor	✓
Clients	✓
Supervisor	✓
Others	☐

Special assessment requirements and what I need to agree with the people concerned:

Supervisor informed of assessment.
Suitable client, tools and products to be available.

Witness testimony sheets.

Schedule for assessment and reviews

Date: *17/2/00*	Date: *10/3/00*	Date: *24/3/00*
Purpose:	Purpose:	Purpose:
Attempt most of performance criteria range for 202.2 and 202.3	*Complete observed and un-observed range statements*	*Complete oral questions*

Candidate signature	Date plan agreed *10/2/97*	Assessor signature
K. Overy		*S. Henderson*

* A blank photocopiable version of this form appears on page 257.

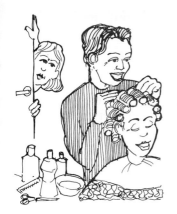

- The **site** is appropriate.
- Suitable **clients** are available.
- **All products, tools and equipment** are **available** and **suitable for the assessment**.

To do

- ■ Re-read the example assessment plan.
- ■ Using the City & Guilds/HTB Level 2 candidate log book:
  - List the performance criteria and range statements that could be assessed for 202.1, 202.2 and 202.3 (Working Safely and Shampoo and Surface-Condition the Hair and Scalp) during a 30-minute assessment on two clients.
  - During your observation of this shampoo process, list the types of products that the candidate could produce as evidence.

Always sit down with your candidate before the assessment and **explain to them exactly what you will be assessing**. Experienced candidates will absorb what you are saying quite quickly, but inexperienced candidates may need you to describe the assessment a couple of times using different phrases and words. A good way of giving encouragement is to say, 'I know you are well practised at this work because you do it all the time in the salon, but I just need to see you do it for assessment purposes today'.

Explain that **all areas of the element** must be assessed in order for them to pass. Always **ask if they have understood what you have said**, giving them the opportunity to ask questions if need be.

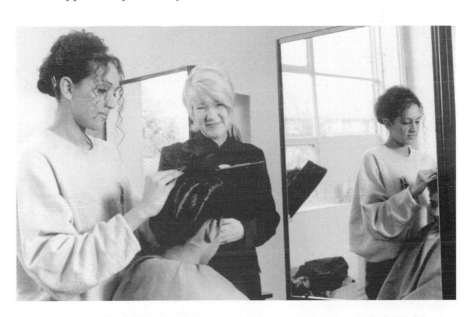

An assessment in progress

4. Gather the evidence from the observation and question the candidate about it

Your candidate could present you with any of the following types of evidence:

- **Natural performance in the workplace.** You record what you see on an observation record sheet (page 187).

185

> **Remember**
>
> You must judge your evidence only against the written criteria. Use only that knowledge, not your own knowledge. For example, shampooing asks for effleurage and rotary massage, not advanced shiatsu massage!

- **Responses to pre-set oral questions and pre-set simulations.** Again, these can be recorded on an observation record sheet. Pre-set oral questions are available only to assessors and should be kept in locked cabinets when not in use (see questioning in Chapter 13).
- **Witness testimonies.** These must be **valid** and **authentic**. They are valid if they refer to the assessment criteria and fall within the relevant time scale (i.e. not ten years ago), and authentic if the signatures match your original specimens and are dated accordingly.

You will need to make up either some **written** or **oral questions** to ask them, to confirm that your candidate has all the knowledge evidence required. See Chapter 13 for more details.

5. Judge the evidence and make your assessment decision

Evidence produced can be not only from practical work, written or oral questions but also from products such as client consultation sheets or record cards.

6. Give your candidate feedback and record it

> **Remember**
>
> Different candidates will have different levels of confidence and experience, so vary your style of feedback accordingly. Always make your feedback constructive and put your candidate at ease by asking 'How did you feel about that assessment?', which encourages them to ask questions and seek advice. Most candidates realise when they have not passed an assessment, so always start by saying something positive, such as 'Your gowning up of the client was fine...' and you have passed the health and safety element, before giving them the bad news: '...but your massage procedure needs a little more practice. How do you think you could improve it?'
>
> Always complete the formative assessments with a written explanation and spend more time in a relaxed manner with under-confident candidates.

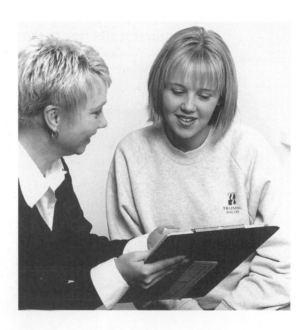

Both successful, i.e. **summative**, and unsuccessful, i.e. **formative**, assessments need to be justified to your candidates through discussion. The recorded results are often written on **Observation Record Sheets** and are always **signed and dated** before being stored. **Summative records** are kept **in the candidate's portfolio**; **formative** records are stored **elsewhere by the candidate**.

Sometimes there may not be enough evidence to make your decision – for instance, the candidate may have wanted to treat a client with dandruff but was unable to because the salon had run out of medicated shampoo.

Observation Record Sheet

206.1 Maintaining safe working methods during hair colouring

(NB part of the performance criteria), 1 observed performance

a)	Have you prepared the client properly?	✓	☐	☐
b)	Have you chosen the correct products, tools and equipment based on the necessary tests and consultation with the client?	✓	☐	☐
c)	Have you prepared the product correctly?	✓	☐	☐
d)	Have you done the necessary hair and skin tests?	✓	☐	☐
e)	Have you checked that your working methods will not endanger either the client or yourself?	✓	☐	☐
f)	Will you be wearing your gloves and dye apron when you are colouring the hair?	☐	☐	☐

Observation 1

Date ___10/03/00___   Candidate signature ___Karen Overy___   Assessor signature ___S Henderson___

Observation 2

Date _____   Candidate signature _____   Assessor signature _____

Observation 3

Date _____   Candidate signature _____   Assessor signature _____

Assessor Comments

(Formative Record Example) No gloves or dye apron were used to apply the semi-permanent colour. The assessment needs to be repeated with protective gloves and dye apron worn.

Example Witness List (including status categories)

Name and contact address	Status	Position*	Elements assessed	Date
Stephanie Linton Connect 2, West Ealing, London W5	2	Salon owner	Witnessed 202.1, 202.2, 202.3, 201.1, 201.2, 201.3	11.3.00

Status categories

Qualified assessor for hairdressing 1
Occupational expert, familiar with standards 2
Occupational expert, not familiar with standards 3
Non-expert 4

* E.g. Senior stylist, college tutor

A Candidate's Work Diary/Witness statement

Name of client	Techniques and methods	Tools and equipment used	Products used	Service provided and how it relates to Performance Criteria	Signature of candidates and witnesses	Unit/element reference
Miss Anderson, 11.3.00	Shampoo and penetrating conditioning treatment for dry hair	Gown, towels, protective capes, bowl, conditioning brush	Shampoo and conditioning treatment for dry hair* * Could be manufacturers' name)	Consultation carried out prior to service starting. I advised Miss Anderson on a suitable shampoo and conditioner for her chemically processed hair, together with a recommendation for 4 further treatments in the salon and products to use at home. I organised the bookings to allow for the extra time involved, and made sure to measure out the exact amount of products. I shampooed using effleurage and rotary movements, and massaged the conditioner using effleurage and petrissage to stimulate the client's natural scalp oils. The conditioner was left on for 10 mins. with extra heat and moisture from the steamer as recommended by the manufacturers. This protective conditioner left the hair tangle-free, soft and shiny, the client was delighted. I then completed the client record card for future treatments on a weekly basis.	S Thomas S Linton	202.1, 202.2, 202.3, 201.1, 201.2, 201.3

Test your knowledge

1. Using the Example Assessment Plan on page 184, describe how you could meet the needs of the following types of candidates.
   - One **experienced** in presenting evidence
   - One **inexperienced** in presenting evidence
   - One with **special assessment** requirements
2. Describe eight different types of acceptable evidence for an assessment and how to select appropriate, efficient methods.
3. Why is important to make an **accurate judgement** by using only the national standards?
4. What is **naturally occurring evidence**, and why is it important for assessment purposes?
5. Describe what **paperwork** you would need for each of the different types of acceptable evidence.
6. Why must the candidate **collect evidence** across the contingency PCs, and how is this done?
7. When would you use a **simulated activity** for assessment, and **who would you consult** if you were unsure of the validity of the simulation?
8. Describe three methods of collecting **knowledge evidence** from an assessment.
9. How do you make sure that assessments are **fair and reliable** (when meeting the candidate's needs) and in line with the national standards?
10. How do the **Equal Opportunities Policy Statements** relate to both you and your candidate?
11. List the different types of **special assessment requirements** and how you could provide for them. Who should you approach for advice?
12. Describe how you could encourage a candidate to take an **active part** in their assessment.
13. Why is it important to make **accurate judgements** against all of the three types of criteria within an element?
14. How could you check that different types of evidence are both **valid and authentic**?
15. Where is the information available about how to administer **pre-set tests**?
16. Describe how to be **unobtrusive** whilst observing an assessment.
17. What types of **difficulty** could occur when making a **judgement of evidence**?
18. Who would you approach **locally** if you had difficulty in judging evidence?
19. Who would you approach **nationally** if you had difficulty in judging evidence?
20. Describe how to ask candidates **oral questions** whilst still maintaining their confidence.
21. How should you give **constructive feedback** to your candidate and maintain their confidence?
22. Why should you encourage your candidate to **ask questions** and **seek advice**?
23. How should you **record** and **process** assessment decisions?

13 Assessing performance (D33)

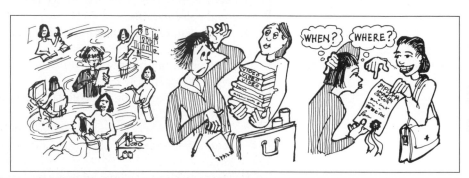

Assessing candidates using differing sources of evidence

Remember

You can use the same candidate that you used for assessing candidate performance for two of the three completed assessment plans you need.

To do

■ Read Chapter 12 and answer the Test Your Knowledge questions before reading this chapter. You will need this understanding first.

What you have to do

1 **Agree an assessment plan with the candidate**
2 **Judge the evidence**
3 **Make your assessment decision using different forms of acceptable evidence and give your candidate feedback**

1. Agree an assessment plan with the candidate

This assessment plan is drawn up in agreement with your candidate and covers at least two elements within the units.

Collecting evidence

You will need to collect **six** of the following sources of evidence from your candidates:

- Observation Record Sheets
- Simulations/role plays
- Projects/assignments
- Oral/written questions
- Witness testimonial (candidate and peer reports)
- Assessment of prior achievements

This evidence needs to be clearly written out so that it can be used for both your own judgement and that of assessors and internal verifiers.

Remember

There are National Standards for assessing oral questions, written questions, projects and assignments.

The standards are contained within the City & Guilds/HTB booklets, Assessment of Essential Knowledge and Understanding, which should be kept in a locked cabinet or room in your assessment centre.

Catering for different needs

Different candidates have different needs. You must find out what type of evidence collection is suitable for your candidate.

- A fully competent and experienced working hairdresser may be almost fully assessed by **natural performance**.
- A candidate undertaking full-time training at a City & Guilds/HTB recognised centre may wish to broaden their education by providing extensive projects and assignments.
- Some candidates may have **special assessment needs** (see Chapter 12).

Always take care to make the best use of both the candidate's time and the resources available. An experienced working hairdresser may not be able to spare the time to produce projects that are not strictly needed.

To do

- Re-read the example assessment plan using the City & Guilds/HTB Level 2 Assessment Record book.
- List the performance criteria, range statements and essential underpinning knowledge that could be assessed for 207.2 (Making Appointments for Services in the Salon) during a 30-minute assessment on two clients.
- During your observation of this process, list the types of acceptable evidence that the candidate could produce.
- Note the differences between experienced candidates, inexperienced candidates and candidates with special assessment needs on a separate sheet of paper.

When you are assessing different sources of evidence, you must be able to confirm that they are all:

- **Valid.** The evidence must refer to all the assessment criteria and City & Guilds/HTB specifications.
- **Authentic.** The handwriting, style of presentation and signatures should match those of the candidate.
- **Current.** The evidence must be up-to-date. A ten-year-old manufacturers' diploma is **not** acceptable.
- **Sufficient.** Every area of the performance criteria, range statements and essential underpinning knowledge should be covered.

You will also need to describe how you would deal with situations where evidence presented has **not** met these key areas. For example:

- **Validity.** If all witness testimonies are signed by a Grade 4 non-expert witness (the candidate's Auntie Maisie, for instance), then more witness testimonies of **higher grades** will need to be produced.
- **Authenticity.** If you suspect that work submitted was not actually done by the candidate, or that signatures have been forged, you will need to take the evidence to the internal verifier for judgement.
- **Current.** If a candidate who is claiming assessment of prior achievements presents a ten-year-old manufacturers' diploma, again the internal verifier will need to second your judgement.
- **Sufficient.** If a candidate has covered all the performance criteria, range statements and essential underpinning knowledge in an element except for two, they will need to be re-assessed to complete those two areas.

An example assessment plan is shown on page 193.

2. Judge the evidence and give your candidate feedback

> **To do**
>
> - Re-read Chapter 12 on judging the evidence and making your assessment decision (page 186).
> - Ask to observe an experienced qualified assessor assessing a candidate performing any of the City & Guilds/HTB Level 2 technical units, such as Unit 202, Shampooing and Conditioning; Unit 203, Styling Hair; Unit 204, Cutting Hair; Unit 205, Perming, Relaxing and Neutralising; Unit 206, Colouring, or Unit 207, Reception.
> - Record whether the assessment was successful (summative) or unsuccessful (formative). Remember not to make any comments that would impede or interfere with the assessment in any way.

Observation Record Sheets (natural performance)

Natural performance, or observing the candidate doing the work, **may not provide enough evidence for the candidate to complete the element**, therefore other **supplementary evidence** may be needed.

If you study the City & Guilds Observation Record Sheets, you will notice that **contingency PCs** are marked with a small asterisk (*). This shows that natural evidence occurs infrequently (such as problems occurring during the perming process), and that supplementary evidence is required.

Supplementary evidence

Simulations/role plays

Simulations are **valid evidence** in the following cases:

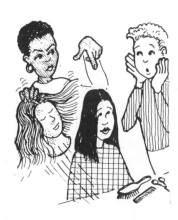

- **When natural evidence occurs infrequently** – e.g. in the case of Level 2 Unit 205 Perming, the performance criteria has a contingency PC relating to problems identified during perming – which could be when incompatibility tests are required – and very few clients have incompatible chemicals already on their hair.
- **When assessing emergency procedures** – e.g. in the case of Level 2 Unit 209 (Health and Safety), which covers hazardous occasions such as fire, flood, bomb alerts, gas leaks, and procedures for dealing with suspicious persons or packages.
- **In situations which might otherwise give rise to an invasion of privacy** – e.g. during a Level 2 Unit 201 assessment of a client with a contagious disorder such as headlice. Here, written evidence, or a role play, are acceptable alternatives.

Simulations are **not** valid evidence, for example, in the case of a long-haired client being unavailable for Unit 203, Dressing Long Hair, and a long-haired tuition head being substituted.

Observed simulations must always be signed and dated by an assessor to confirm that it is a **valid** and acceptable piece of evidence.

> **To do**
>
> - Look through the Level 2 observation record sheets and find two other occasions when it might be necessary to use simulations or role plays as supplementary evidence.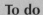

Example Assessment Plan*

Candidate's name	*Sharon Stevens*
Assessor	*S Henderson*
Unit no. and title	*207. Reception*
Element no. and title	*207.3 Handling Client Payments*
Approximate timing of assessment	*30 mins natural performance*
	15 mins oral questions + feedback

Evidence to be presented

Natural performance in the workplace	✓	Records of prior achievement	☐
Responses to oral questions	✓	Reports from supervisors in workplaces	✓
Written projects and assignments	☐	Simulated work activities	☐
Review of written records e.g. client record cards	☐		
Completed assessment question papers	☐		

Details

1. Natural performance in the workplace
Covering performance criteria and range statements cash and cheque

2. Responses to oral questions
Relating to line management, salon security, consequences of incorrect payment handling, effective communication – both verbal and non-verbal, message reporting, operating the salon appointment systems, salon services – costs and durations, retail products

Covering types of payment procedure, invalid and fraudulent payments

4. Reports from supervisors in workplaces
Complete one assessment (unobserved by assessor) with witness testimonies signed by work placement supervisor covering supplementary evidence such as low levels of change.

People involved in my assessment

Assessor	✓
Clients	✓
Supervisor	✓
Others	☐

Special assessment requirements and what I need to agree with the people concerned

Supervisor informed of assessment.
Assessment booked – cash shortages.
Witness testimony sheets.

Schedule for assessment and review

Date: *17/3/00*	Date: *3/4/00*	Date: *4/4/00*
Purpose: *Assessment of 207.3 pc's and oral questions*	Purpose: *Supplementary evidence witness statements completed*	Purpose: *Feedback of completed elements 207.3*
Candidate signature	Date plan agreed	Assessor signature
S. Stevens	*3/3/00*	*S. Henderson*

* A blank photocopiable version of this form appears on page 257.

Assignments

City & Guilds have pre-set assignments that are specified for the following units: Unit 203, Styling Hair; Unit 204, Cutting; Unit 209, Health and Safety; Unit 210, Barbering; Unit 212 Cutting Men's Facial Hair; and Unit 213, Blow Drying Men's Hair.

You must make sure that your candidate has a **clear understanding** of the assignment and the knowledge and understanding required. A good way to do this is to ask your candidate to explain the written project or assignments back to you, **using their own words**.

Assignments may be **hand-written or typed**. The length is often specified, such as four sheets of A4. Candidates are also encouraged to include evidence generated as part of their practical performance, such as:

- Client record cards
- Photographs of hairstyles they have produced
- Drawings
- Illustrations of tools and equipment used for specific techniques
- Stock record sheets

Other forms of evidence may also be used for illustration purposes. For example:

- Manufacturers' instructions for various products
- Manufacturers' leaflets and product brochures
- Health and Safety leaflets

There is no harm in candidates including additional information if it helps them to understand the subject. On the other hand, they are only required to cover the knowledge and understanding specified.

To do

- Write up your own answer guides for the following projects/assignments (which currently do not have specified City & Guilds/HTB answer guides):
  - Unit 203, Styling Hair
  - Unit 204, Cutting
  - Unit 209, Health and Safety
  - Unit 210, Barbering
  - Unit 212, Cutting Men's Facial Hair
  - Unit 213, Blow Drying Men's Hair
  Check your answers with your internal verifier or a fellow assessor.

Questioning

You can ask **oral** questions or set **written** questions. Most are **pre-set** by City & Guilds/HTB, but you may have to make up some of your own to suit your own **salon policy** dictates.

Oral questions

Here are some examples of oral questions related to a particular salon policy:

To do

■ Re-read Chapter 11 on asking oral questions (pages 174–175).

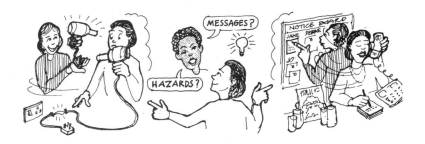

Remember

Always brief your candidate fully directly before an assessment. Remember that the assessment plan may have been made days or weeks beforehand.

Explain what you will be questioning on – e.g. health and safety, oral questions relating to colouring – and why you will be asking those questions. For example, if no problems occurred during the perming process, you would need to ask the candidate what they would have done if problems had occurred.

Q. 'How do you record and pass on messages in your salon?'
A. 'Either hand the message directly to the person or pin to the noticeboard behind the reception desk if the person is unavailable. You must always make sure you notify the person about the message as soon as possible.'
Q. 'At what stage would you refer a hazard to the relevant person?'
A. 'When the hazard could be a danger to other people – for example, a damaged electrical flex.'

Never lead the candidates when asking questions – for example, by saying, 'Look at that damaged electrical flex, it looks rather dangerous. Who should you be speaking to about it?'

Remember

All written questions and answer guides must be kept in a securely locked cabinet for internal and external verification procedures.

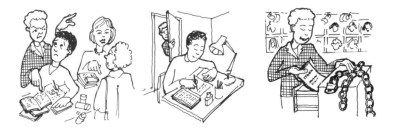

Written questions
City & Guilds/HTB have pre-set written questions with answer guides available to assessors.

To do

■ Study your centre's City & Guilds/HTB Written Assessment Header Sheets. Find out:
  – What parts your candidate completes and which parts you complete
  – Where the assessment co-ordinator signs and where you sign
  – What your centre number is
  – How to record correct and incorrect answers
  Note that the assessment co-ordinator and the assessor may not necessarily be the same person.

Remember

When marking written assessment you are looking for the correct answers. Do not take marks off for incorrect answers.

If your candidate has clearly failed one or two questions, then they must wait for two weeks and then resit those two questions again. If necessary, they can resit any failed questions again after another two weeks.

If your candidate is still unsuccessful then they must wait for two months before taking the whole written assessment again.

These questions must be given to the candidate soon after the completion of a successful natural performance assessment. The candidate needs to have access to a **quiet area** where they will not be interrupted during this written assessment. A busy salon reception desk is **not** a suitable area.

The written questions must be supervised by an assessment co-ordinator who signs to confirm that the assessment was valid – i.e. that no reference materials were used or that the candidate did not collaborate with others to produce the answers.

Header sheets must always be attached to the completed written test papers and filled in correctly.

City & Guilds/HTB have strict rules about the implementation of written assessments. Each assessment has a **time limit** (which may average 4–5 minutes per question).

Types of written questions

Written questions can take many different forms:

1. Short answer
For example:

Q. 'Name the part of the hair that is affected by a temporary colour.'
A. 'The cuticle scale.'

2. Incomplete sentences
For example:

Q. 'Professional hairdressers always pick up and hold their scissors with their _____ and _____ _____ .'
A. 'Thumb and third finger.'

3. Selection of correct answers from a list
For example:

Q. Underline two infectious diseases from the list below:
Seborrhoea   Impetigo   Sebaceous cyst
Psoriasis   Pediculosis capitis   Alopecia areata
A. Impetigo, Pediculosis capitis

4. Diagrams
For example: Label the following diagrams:

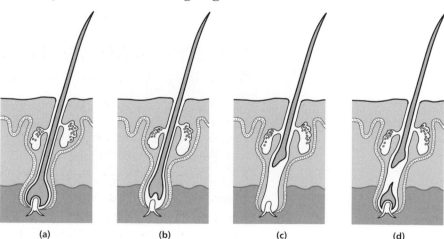

(a)   (b)   (c)   (d)

A. (a) Anagen active growth (1–7 years); (b) Catagen breakdown and change (two weeks); (c) Telogen resting stage (3–4 months); (d) Anagen regrowth.

5. Completion of tables

For example: Fill in the spaces on the following table (completed table below):

Q: Hydrogen Peroxide Dilutions			
Volume of hydrogen peroxide	Parts of hydrogen peroxide	Parts of distilled water	Volume
60	_____ +	_____ =	40
60	_____ +	_____ =	30
60	_____ +	_____ =	20
60	_____ +	_____ =	10
40	_____ +	_____ =	30
40	_____ +	_____ =	20
40	_____ +	_____ =	10
30	_____ +	_____ =	20
30	_____ +	_____ =	10
20	_____ +	_____ =	10

A: Hydrogen Peroxide Dilutions			
Volume of hydrogen peroxide	Parts of hydrogen peroxide	Parts of distilled water	Volume
60	2 +	1 =	40
60	1 +	1 =	30
60	1 +	2 =	20
60	1 +	5 =	10
40	3 +	1 =	30
40	1 +	1 =	20
40	1 +	3 =	10
30	2 +	1 =	20
30	1 +	2 =	10
20	1 +	1 =	10

Witness testimonies (candidate and peer reports)

Here are some examples of different types of candidate and peer reports:

- **Candidate work diary/witness statement** (see worked example in Chapter 12, page 188)
- **Messages** taken by telephone or in person (see below)
- **Client record cards** (see below)
- Annotated **stock record sheets** (see page 198)
- **Candidate appraisals** and their responses to these
- **Action plans** (e.g. page 200). These are useful to guide the candidate as to how much they can achieve within a specified period of time.

Example of a message
taken

Telephone Message

From *Mrs Brown*   Date *4/4*

To   *Caroline*   Time *2.30 pm*

Caller's tel. no. *0012578*

Message

She'll be 45 minutes late.

Can you call her back?

Hair Colour Record Card

Client name _____	Natural hair colour _____
Address _____	Texture _____
_____	Condition _____
Daytime tel. no. _____	_____
Skin test _____ Date _____	Name of operator _____

Record of application

Date _____

Type _____

Colour _____

Hydrogen Peroxide _____

Development   *Method* _____

                 Time _____

Application Special Notes _____

Comb through _____

After treatment _____

Result   *Required* _____

            Obtained _____

Stylist _____

Stock Record Sheet

	Salon Products	P Code	Pack Size	Max. Level	Min. Level	Stock	Order	Del'd.
1.0	Natural purifying cleanser	P1050	1					
1.8	Colour vitalising cleanser	P1057	1					
1.9	Perm energising cleanser	P1058	1					
1.2	Replenishing cleanser	P1051	1					
1.3	Ultimate volume cleanser	P1052	1					
1.C	Active cleanser	P1053	1					
1.4	Clarifying cleanser	P1054	1					
1.7	Active balancing cleanser	P1056	1					
1.6	Soothing Derma Cleanser	P1055	1					

Candidate Appraisal Form*

Name _____

Date _____

	Supervisor's Grading		Supervisor's Grading
Attendance	☐	Cutting	☐
Punctuality	☐	Setting	☐
Attitude to work	☐	Blow Drying	☐
Attitude to group/other staff	☐	Perming	☐
Attitude to clients	☐	Colouring	☐
Personal presentation	☐		
Written assignment marks	☐		

Candidate response

_____

_____

Signature _____

Supervisor's comments

_____

_____

Signature _____

Grading: **A** – Excellent **B** – Very Good **C** – Good **D** – Average **E** – Poor

---

To do
■ Make up your own examples of worked candidate and peer reports and check with your centre's internal verifier to see if they could be valid pieces of supplementary evidence.

Remember

The candidate's competence must be current, and the evidence must be authentic and verifiable.

For example, a letter from the candidate's employer saying that they helped with a hairdressing show would not be acceptable.

Assessment of prior achievement

If your candidate can produce any **evidence of past achievements**, then they may be able to use this as another type of valid evidence. For example, a Level 3 candidate may have a recent manufacturers' Advanced Colour Diploma, or have **past demonstrations of competence** such as planning evidence or perhaps a video of a hairdressing show put on by their salon. On page 201 is an example of a Level 3 candidate's piece of verifiable evidence towards Unit 11, Demonstrating and Instructing.

* A full-size photocopiable version of this form appears on page 246.

Candidate Practical Action Plan*

Name	*Tracey Emery*
Start date	*9/9/00*

Date	*24/9/00*
Target elements	*202.1, 202.2, 202.3 Shampooing & Conditioning* *201.1 Client Consultation*

Candidate signature

T. Emery

Target date	*17/11/00*
Comments	*I have one year's work experience in a salon and need to reinforce my underpinning knowledge*

Assessor signature

S. Henderson

Date	_____
Target elements	_____
Target date	_____
Comments	_____

Candidate signature

Assessor signature

This type of evidence needs to be checked carefully to make sure that it is not outdated – techniques, products and equipment may have changed. Evidence of prior achievements may also be **harder to gather** because of time lapses, and may need to be **endorsed by witnesses**.

When these difficulties occur, you must always advise your candidate that it may be easier for them to simply reproduce the evidence.

Your centre will often employ someone who has a **D36 (APL Advisor) Certificate**, which means they are qualified to assess prior learning achievements. This person will be able to advise you if you are unsure about the validity of the evidence.

On page 202 is a completed sample APL evidence summary sheet which you may use as a guide.

---

3. Make your assessment decision using different forms of acceptable evidence and give your candidate feedback

Observation Record Sheets (natural performance)

See Chapter 12.

---

* A full-size photocopiable version of this form appears on page 255.

An example of verifiable
evidence of past
competence

26th October 1999

TO WHOM IT MAY CONCERN

I would like to confirm that Kirsten Harjette was
employed at Uxbridge College from 1997 to 1999 to teach
Hairdressing at NVQ Level 1 and 2.

She has covered Level 3, Unit 11, Demonstrating and
Instructing Students, at both her levels on many
occasions to a satisfactory standard, and has been
witnessed by me as her line manager.

Yours faithfully,

J. Chivell

Ms. J. Chivell
Course Team Leader Hairdressing

> **Remember**
>
> Summative decisions mean
> that the candidate has passed.
>
> Formative decisions mean the
> candidate has not yet passed.

> **Remember**
>
> Your assessment decisions
> must be consistent. If an
> answer guide is not supported
> by City & Guilds/HTB, then
> write up your own and check
> it with the internal verifier
> before marking.

> **Remember**
>
> If your candidate has special
> assessment needs – e.g. is
> recognised by the internal and
> external verifiers as a
> Statemented Dyslexic – then
> you must seek clarification of
> your assessment decision.

Simulations/role plays

Summative example
A short **written description of an incompatibility test** procedure may be
used as supplementary evidence (see page 26).

Formative example
Lack of written evidence or oral questions is an example of insufficient
evidence.

Projects/assignments

Summative example
A cutting (Unit 204) project containing the following:

Four illustrations of current fashion looks

- Including references to:
  - Two one-length and two layered looks
  - One one-length look with a fringe, one layer cut with a graduation
- An explanation of cutting techniques – club cutting, scissor- and
  clipper-over-comb, thinning with scissors or razor and freehand –
  including how to produce each look and how they are used to achieve
  the overall effect.

Example APL Evidence Summary Sheet*

| Candidate's name: | *Kirsten Harjette* | | Award title: | *City & Guilds/HTB Hairdressing Level 3* |
| Assessor's name: | *Stephanie Henderson* | | | |

Unit or element claimed	Listing of experience	References and CV	Product evidence	Certificates and awards
Unit 11, Facilitate learning through Demonstration and Instruction	*Training junior staff at "Stage Door" salon from 1995–1997* *Teaching and assessing hair-dressing Levels 1 & 2 candidates at Uxbridge College 1997–1999*	*Reference from "Stage Door" salon* *CV stating all qualifications, training and experience*	*Lesson plans incorporating demonstration techniques to candidates at Uxbridge College*	*City & Guilds/HTB Level 2 Hairdressing* *Wella "Train the Trainer" Diploma* *C&G D32 & D33 certificates*

Interview notes	Other evidence	Top-up training needed	Sufficient valid evidence
Kirsten had a good understanding of the performance criteria range statements of Unit 11. However, she needs to provide details of Health & Safety legislation & good practice	*Witness testimony from Jan Chivell, Course Team Leader & Line Manager at Uxbridge College*	*Kirsten needs to attend the lecture relating to "Demonstrating & Instructing Learners" to clarify the Health & Safety requirements of the unit*	*A small project regarding Health & Safety legislation & good practice during demonstrating & instructing candidates to be produced by 7.5.00*

Candidate's signature	Date assessment plan agreed
K. Harjette	*4/4/00*

Assessor's signature	Date of assessment
S. Henderson	*7/5/00*

* A blank photocopiable version of this form appears on page 254.

Example of Feedback Given to an Inexperienced Candidate*

NVQ Level 2 Cutting Project
Unit 4

Candidate name   David Darling

Date   7/5/00

Assessor's comments

A very good project, David. It is beautifully illustrated and clearly written. However, you just need to include a little more about how freehand cutting could be used on your one length cut with a fringe.

You also need to be clearer about the differences between club cutting and graduating

---

Assessor's name   S.Henderson

Assessor's signature   *S.Henderson*

Student signature   *D. Durling*

Passed/Referred

* This is an example of constructive feedback giving different types of advice

---

- A list of the circumstances in which the hair would be cut wet or dry

Formative example
The candidate has not covered some areas in the project specification or has provided incorrect explanations.

Oral/written questions

Oral questions
Summative example (Unit 207, Reception):

Q. 'What action would you take if a payment discrepancy occurred?'
A. 'Refer to the lecturer in charge of the practical class (e.g. if the client queried her bill). If the change given was incorrect, it would need to be rechecked.'

Formative example (Unit 202, Shampooing and Conditioning):

Q. 'What are the range of shampoos, surface conditioners and conditioning treatments available for use with different hair and scalp conditions?'
A. 'Medicated shampoos and herbal anti-oxy conditioners.'

There is not sufficient evidence in this answer.

Written questions
Summative example:

Q. 'Name the part of the hair that is affected by a temporary colour.'
A. 'The cuticle scale'

Formative example:

Q. 'Professional hairdressers always pick up and hold their scissors with their _____ and _____ finger.'

A. 'Thumb and first finger'

This must be marked as **incorrect**, and the candidate **needs to know** that this question was answered incorrectly.

Witness testimonies/candidate and peer reports

Summative example: A correctly completed candidate work diary/witness statement as in Chapter 12, page 188.

Formative example: An incomplete message taken by telephone. For example:

This is an example of a situation where you need to encourage your candidate to ask why you have given a formative assessment. The candidate needs to know that the message should have been completed by adding the person the message was for, the time and the caller's telephone number.

Assessment of prior achievements

This is often used for candidates who are **experienced in presenting evidence**.

Summative example: A letter confirming a past demonstration of competence (see page 201).

Formative example: An outdated manufacturers' diploma, such as a 1960s Tepid Perm.

Giving feedback on a combination of evidence

Often a candidate may submit **differing sources of evidence** to be assessed, not only by you but also by other assessors.

> **To do**
>
> - Re-read the Example Assessment Plan (page 193) and name the four different types of evidence that may be presented.

To check that a candidate has completed all three types of relevant criteria, i.e. the performance criteria, the range statements and the underpinning knowledge, all the evidence must be **valid**, **authentic**, **current** and **sufficient**. Therefore you must check the **content**, the **signatures** and **dates** and the **sufficiency of the evidence** before both you and the candidate sign and date to confirm that the element is complete.

Recording and processing assessment decisions

The **summative** copies are kept in the **candidates' portfolios**, the **formative** copies are kept by the **candidates themselves**.

Observation Record Sheets (natural performance), including the performance criteria, range statements and underpinning knowledge areas, are ticked, comments written in, signed and dated.

Summative copies of the following should be completed, signed and dated by the assessor and candidate, and filed in the candidate's portfolio:

- **Simulations/role plays**
- **Projects/assignments**
- **Witness testimonies/candidate peer reports**
- **Assessment of prior achievements**

In the case of **oral questions**, you need to record which questions you have asked the candidates on the Observation Record Sheets.

For **written questions**, both summative and formative questions and answers should always be kept in a locked cabinet or room.

> **Test your knowledge**
>
> 1 List the **six different methods** for collecting evidence.
> 2 How could you find which **method of evidence** is relevant for a particular element?
> 3 Give one example of a **valid** piece of evidence for each.
> 4 Describe a type of candidate who would require **cost-effective** and **efficient selection of evidence**.
> 5 Why is an **assessment plan** needed?
> 6 How should you prepare an assessment plan that incorporates **authentic choice** for your candidates?
> 7 Why should you use only **City & Guilds/HTB specified pre-set** oral and written questions, projects and assignments?
> 8 Describe the procedure for assessing candidates with the following type of special assessment needs:
>   - A **hearing-impaired** candidate
>   - A registered **dyslexic** candidate
>
> **Continued**

205

Test your knowledge *continued*

9 Describe how to give **constructive feedback** to a candidate who seems nervous, or lacking in confidence or experience during both formative and summative assessments (see Chapter 12).

10 How should you make **fair, reliable and consistent judgements** of your candidate's evidence if you are unclear about City & Guilds/HTB answer guides?

11 What are the **three** types of **relevant criteria** in an element?

12 How could you check the **authenticity** of a candidate's evidence?

13 Describe the correct methods for **administering** City & Guilds/HTB **pre-set** oral, and written questions and simulations.

14 Describe how to be **unobtrusive** whilst observing an assessment.

15 Who should you approach **locally** and **nationally** if you have difficulty in judging evidence?

16 Describe how to encourage your candidate to **ask questions and seek advice** (see Chapter 11).

17 How should you **record** and **process** each of the different methods of evidence?

18 How is the candidate **verified**?

14 Teamwork

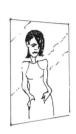
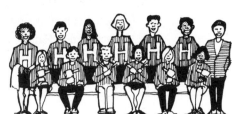
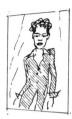

The salon team

Remember

Staff **personnel** may be **full time** or **part time**, **permanent** or **temporary**, **internal** or **external** and **paid** or **voluntary** – they all work for your organisation.

Who are the team members in a salon? They could be:

- Other trainees
- Junior and senior stylists
- Supervisors
- Managers
- Others working in the salon such as receptionists, beauty therapists, people on work experience, cleaning staff or catering staff
- Voluntary, unpaid helpers such as work placement students from colleges and schools

Salons vary in size, so there may be just you and a few other staff in a small salon, or you could be part of a medium-to-large salon of 4–20 people, or even part of a large chain of salons employing hundreds of hairdressers. Wherever you work, you will need to not only do your own work well, but to help and support the rest of the team in an enthusiastic and pleasant manner.

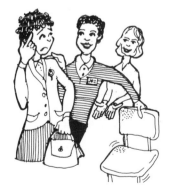

Managing your own workload

Line management
On page 208 is an example of a line management chart, which you might like to use as a model when drawing up your own.

Lines of management and each person's limit of authority are important, especially when dealing with **client complaints**, **staff discipline** and **appraisals**.

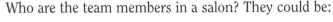

To do

■ Draw up your own line management chart for your salon.

As a manager or supervisor you need to know:

- Your **defined area of responsibility**
- How to take **decisions** and **manage budgets** within specified limited opportunities – e.g. sending staff on training courses

Line Management Chart*

Name	Position	Experience and qualification	Limits of authority
Kevin	Owner	20 years' hairdressing; D32, D33, D34; Level II Hairdressing; C&G Ladies Hairdressing.	Preparing job descriptions. All salon finances. All team problems. Rules and regulations. Health and Safety. Firing staff.
Kirsten	Manager	16 years' hairdressing; D32, D33; Level 3 Hairdressing; New Zealand hairdressing qualification.	Allocation of staff roles and responsibilities. All technical problems. Interviewing and appointing new staff. Disciplinary procedures. Work allocations. Reports to owner.
Jan	Artistic Director	16 years' hairdressing; Master Craftsman; Level 3 Hairdressing; C&G Ladies & Gents' Hairdressing.	Organisation of salon shows, promotions and photographic work. Reports to Manager.
Antonella	Senior Stylist	12 years' hairdressing; D32, D33, D34; Level 2 Hairdressing; Level 3 Hairdressing.	Staff trainer. Reports to Manager.
Natasha	Stylist	8 years' hairdressing; Level 2 Hairdressing; Level 3 Hairdressing ongoing.	Reports to Manager or Senior Stylist.
Nicola	Receptionist	5 years as receptionist; Qualified in secretarial skills.	Responsible for stock control and appointments. Reports to Manager.
Claire	Junior Stylist	3 years, 2 years' training; Level 2 Hairdressing.	Reports to Senior Stylist.
Darren	Junior	18 months' ongoing Level 2 hairdressing.	Reports to Senior Stylist.
Andrew	Junior	6 months' ongoing Level 2 hairdressing.	Reports to Senior Stylist.
Jenny	P/T Saturday Junior	6 months' ongoing Level I hairdressing.	Reports to Senior Stylist.

* A blank photocopiable version of this form appears on page 256.

- How to **use resources effectively** to achieve specific results – e.g. setting time aside to appraise staff to improve their capabilities and increase business for the salon
- How to **allocate work** to all staff personnel

Leadership

Good leaders must have an understanding of how to build a strong team that can work harmoniously and effectively. To do this a leader must have abilities in a number of areas.

Communication

Many clients return to a salon because it has a **good atmosphere** and the staff are always happy and cheerful. Tension or bad atmospheres in the salon can result in lost clients and poor working relationships.

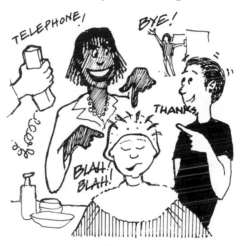

Continuous improvement

A leader will inspire continuous improvement in the staff by **identifying training needs** through individual and team appraisals.

Information handling

Staff feedback regarding client services may be obtained in several ways, by:

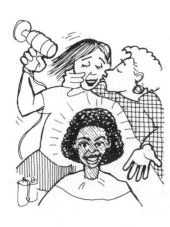

- General **discussion** – **informally** in the staff rest room during breaks, or **formally** during staff meetings.
- In a **written** form, either through **staff appraisals** (see page 218) or by **brainstorming** during a staff (or team) meeting. Brainstorming sessions are where everyone throws out suggestions which are all written up on a flip chart or noted down, after which they can be analysed and discussed. This information can be itemised and used for future reference.

Involvement and motivation

Everyone works for money, which is the strongest motivating force. However, you will have noticed that **some people work harder than others**! Motivating factors depend on people's age and where they are in life:

- Mature stylists with their own established clientele may be quite satisfied with just doing their jobs well and see no point in progressing further.
- A young recently qualified stylist may be very ambitious and wish to participate in every training course, promotion, show or photographic session available.

Organisational context

Before you can allocate and supervise another person's work you must find out from your immediate manager exactly what you are allowed to do (i.e. what work is within the **limits of your authority**). For example, you may feel it would be helpful to carry out a complete salon stock-take, but your manager may have delegated that responsibility to a new manufacturer's company representative.

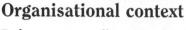

To do

- Before you start to allocate work in the salon, make **two lists** of all the tasks that need to be done. Make one list for **technical** work such as perms, tints, cuts, etc., and one for **non-technical** work such as reception, salon stock and cleaning duties.
- Once you have made up your lists you need to decide who does what. There are several criteria you must bear in mind:
  - **The competence requirements of the work**. For example, a new product from the manufacturer is best trialled on a less busy working day, when staff have time to go through the instructions thoroughly.
  - **The competence requirements of the individuals**. For example, it is not a good idea to allocate foil highlighting to a junior until you have seen their work on a model.
  - **The existing work commitments of the individuals**. For example, a stylist with a full Saturday clientele would not take kindly to being asked to fit in a wedding party on that day!

Training and development

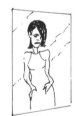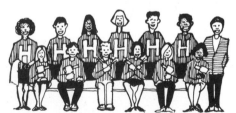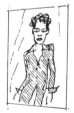

To support your staff in practical terms you could:

- **Assist salon staff with their technical work** either by offering practical help (e.g. winding their perms or helping with foil highlights) or by providing technical advice (e.g. talking through a colour correction problem).
- **Participate in staff training sessions** – for example, by either offering to do a demonstration or by planning ahead and rescheduling appointments so that training can take place.
- **Organise a salon promotion** – using your initiative, you could ask your existing manufacturing company to provide an in-house seminar to train staff in the use of new products or equipment.

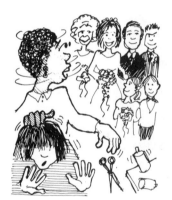

Remember

Most people have their general job description already, therefore you must allocate work around those descriptions.

Remember

Managing or supervising others is a learned skill. You need to understand and apply the principles behind it.

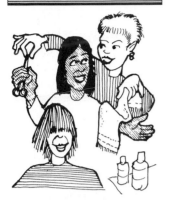

Acting assertively

During conflict situations you need to **state your own views and position clearly**. A **knowledge** of both the **salon rules** (see page 106) and **job descriptions** helps to clear up any discrepancies.

You will also need to maintain your beliefs, commitment and efforts when there are set-backs and opposition.

Promoting harmony in your team

Generally team harmony is provided by:

- Staff and management accepting and giving feedback in a positive way
- Staff being competent within their job – i.e. not being allocated work which is beyond their skills and capabilities
- Staff supporting each other as part of a team – i.e. not just relying on juniors to help out when necessary, but using their initiative to help each other all the time

Building teams

As a leader you will need to

- **Make time** to help and support everyone
- Give **encouragement** to stimulate others, and to **motivate them**, whatever their capabilities
- Evaluate and **give everyone feedback** to help improve their future performances
- Use your **authority** and power **fairly** – don't have favourites!
- Keep everyone **informed** about whatever **progress** has been made and what **future plans** are happening
- Invite **everyone to contribute** to future work developments
- **Set** achievable and challenging **objectives** and **goals**

Effective communication

You can communicate helpfully with your staff by:

- **Offering your support verbally** – e.g. by helping with technical advice or by praising their efforts
- **Providing practical assistance when necessary** – e.g. by attending to one of their clients if they are behind with their work schedule
- **Listening actively** – by asking questions and rephrasing the person's statements to check mutual understanding e.g. 'what do you understand by a haircut over the ear?'
- **Identifying what information is needed** by the person you are speaking to e.g. 'do you need to refresh your hair colouring knowledge or develop some new advanced techniques?'

If you wish to communicate messages to staff, you need to decide:

- **Who needs to receive the message**. If it is everyone, then a staff meeting may be difficult to organise if everyone works on different times and days. Perhaps a social staff meeting might be more convenient?
- **How to communicate the message** – i.e. verbally or in writing? If the

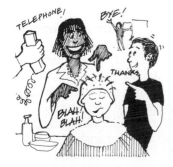

211

message is **verbal**, you will need to check that the receiver has understood and will action the message. If the message is **written**, you will need to make sure that it reaches the right person and is understood by them. Remember also that people communicate all the time by using **body language** – e.g. someone who avoids eye contact with you may not necessarily be accepting the message you are sending.

You must always be **sensitive** when giving and receiving messages or information to your staff, and check that they know what they have to do and how to do it.

Decision making

In the same way that all hairdressers have to project a professional image to their clients and need to give clients their full attention, you, as a supervisor or manager, must **never allow salon problems to interfere with your salon management**. Remember, the professional image of your salon is at stake. All problems must be dealt with in a calm, considered way.

Use your **own experience** and **look at all the evidence** before making a decision.

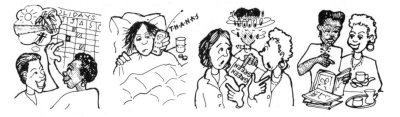

Personnel issues (i.e. difficulties keeping up with scheduled appointments)

Staff are the salon's major resource, so you must plan carefully and make sure information is passed on to those who need it:

- **Staff holidays:** Not only must the clients be rescheduled to suitable members of staff, but you must have a **written staff holiday rota** so that you know in advance if two or more people are going to be away at the same time.
- **Staff sickness:** Always implement a **staff sickness procedure**, e.g. a statement should be written into job descriptions, requiring members of staff who are ill to notify the salon **as soon as it opens for business**. This will enable you to reschedule all the clients **before the start of the working day**.

Technical problems (i.e. lack of assistance from team members)

As a supervisor or manager you will often be asked for **advice and support**. Think back and remember how you felt when you had to wind your first perm and all the perm rods kept falling out and you didn't know which perm lotion to choose! Before giving any advice, take the member of staff to a **quiet area away from the client** and explain clearly and slowly what you think they should do. Always ask them to repeat it back to you by saying 'Now exactly which colour and peroxide strength did we decide on?' This will ensure that they have completely understood your instructions and will reinforce their confidence.

Emergency situations

Health and safety

All salons must have a **Health and Safety Policy**, including details of **evacuation procedures** in the event of fire, flood, gas leak, bomb alert or suspicious packages. Careful policy procedures are needed for all of these disruptions to services, and must not only be explained to new staff but regularly confirmed with existing staff.

First aid procedures

First aid procedures in the case of major or minor accidents or illnesses **must** be understood and carried out by all the staff. Most large organisations have a qualified first aider in attendance, and it is a good idea to have a qualified first aider in any salon.

General salon matters

If everyone in your salon has a written job description, laid out in the same way as a line management chart, then it will be very clear to them exactly what everyone's job role is. For example, in an emergency whose job is it to evacuate the salon?

To do

- If you were absent from the salon through sickness, because you were on holiday or because you were attending a training course, name and inform the person in your salon responsible for:
  - Client complaints
  - Staff discipline
  - Rescheduling appointments (due to staff absences)
  - Obtaining emergency stock
  - Dealing with technical problems
  - Salon emergency procedures

Improving the salon

Remember

Praise is an excellent motivator.

Telling someone off is a negative motivating force.

Salon services need to be improved continually, not only for **profitability** but to **inform**, **motivate**, **train** and **develop the staff**. Managers and supervisors implement the principles of good practice by identifying needs, planning and contributing to activities and assessing the results.

To motivate staff you need to set them goals, either individually or as a team. However, the goals must be:

- **Specific** – in other words, the goal must be clear. You should not simply say to a junior 'Go and improve'. Improve what? You should say for example 'You need to improve your perm winding time.'
- **Achievable** – the goal must be achievable by that person. For example, 'You need to improve your perm winding time. It took you $2\frac{1}{2}$ hours today; try doing it in 2 hours next time.'
- **Measurable** – The goal must be measured either by you or the person involved, e.g. 'Look at the clock and note when you started winding that perm, so you can see how long it took you.'
- **Acceptable** – The junior must want to accept the task. For example,

before attempting perming again, they might prefer to concentrate on setting and try to achieve a reasonable time for putting rollers in a set.

The staff group could be equally motivated by setting a salon team goal such as increasing your client base by doing a show. The resulting increase in profits would benefit everyone.

Developing the salon (team objectives)

One of the best ways to discover how to improve your services is by asking your clients.

There are several ways of encouraging client feedback. These include using open-ended questions, having a suggestion box or a client comment box or using a client questionnaire (See Chapter 1). An example of a client questionnaire appears on page 215.

If using a questionnaire, remember to hand your client a pen or pencil and something to lean on towards the end of the service when politely asking them to fill it in.

It is important to analyse this information regularly and act upon it to improve your salon services.

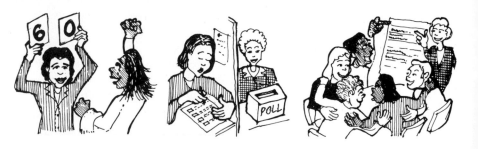

Staff development (individual objectives and aspirations)

Appraisals

Appraisal systems enable both you and the staff to discuss what **development** is needed for both the **salon organisation** and for **them individually**. By setting objectives and goals together you can recommend the best way to achieve them.

A **pre-appraisal** allows for consideration regarding 'where you are now', an appraisal looks at 'where you are going', and an **appraisal review** enables you to look at 'whether you have achieved your goals or objectives'.

Identifying staff needs

A pre-appraisal questionnaire given to staff a few weeks before an appraisal will identify staff development needs and can be presented at an appropriate time during appraisals.

During the completion of the pre-appraisal questionnaire staff will have an opportunity to contribute to their own development needs – for example,

Client Questionnaire*

In our salon **you** the client are the most **important person**. We would therefore like to improve our service to you and would appreciate a few moments of your time to complete this simple questionnaire.

Date _____

Service required _____

Area where you live _____

Your age group 15–25 / 35–45 / 45–60 / 60+ *(please circle)*

What time of day did you attend? 9 am–12 pm / 12 pm–2 pm / 2 pm–6 pm / 6 pm–9 pm *(please circle)*

Was your service… Excellent/Good/Average/Poor *(please circle)*

Were you given a free consultation? Yes/No

Was the salon up to the required standard of cleanliness? Yes/No

What was the attitude of the staff that attended to you? Excellent/Good/Average/Poor *(please circle)*

Did you have to wait for any part of your service? Yes/No

(if applicable) Was the waiting time acceptable to you? Yes/No

Are you happy with the quality of service offered at our salon? Yes/No

Do you consider our salon gives good value for money? Yes/No

Are you dissatisfied with any part of the service offered? Yes/No

If yes, briefly describe what was wrong _____

_____

Would you like any additional hairdressing or beauty Yes/No
services offered in the salon?

If yes, please describe. _____

If you are a new client, will you return to us? Yes/No

If no, why not? _____

If you are a regular client, what is it that keeps you coming to us? _____

Is there any particular member of staff you find outstanding? Yes/No

If yes, who is it? _____

Please place the questionnaire in the box by reception as you leave

Many thanks

* A full-size photocopiable version of this form appears on pages 247 and 248.

Pre-Appraisal Questionnaire*

Name of Appraisee *Rachel Davies*
Job Title *Senior Stylist*

Current work & responsibilities

Staff trainer
Attends to clients
Long hair specialist

Objectives achieved and outstanding objectives

Achieved Planning and reviews of model nights for juniors
Long hair training sessions
Outstanding objectives – to review and prepare a report on client questionnaires

Which areas of work are you least satisfied with?

My time management

What topics or issues would you like to discuss?

To include hair extensions as a new salon service
To attend a time management course

Development Needs

What skills do you feel need to be developed further?

Feedback and reviews to juniors on their training during model nights

What particular training do you require?

Training in the application of both synthetics and real hair extension
Time management training

Name *RACHEL DAVIES* Signature *R Davies* Date *3/11/99*

* A blank photocopiable version of this form appears on page 249.

they will be able to reflect on both past and future training. A full appraisal needs time – usually 1½–2 hours in a quiet area, with no interruptions, and gives both the appraisee and the appraiser time to consider what **development needs** are **relevant and realistic** and take account of team and **organisational constraints** (such as **salon policies**, **time** and **money**).

The individual development needs can then be considered against the needs of the other staff. You may then decide, perhaps, that a specialist giving 'in-house' training to all staff will be more cost-effective than individual training courses.

To do

■ Look at the example of a completed pre-appraisal form, then list which developments apply to team objectives and which apply to individual aspirations.

Integrating individual and team objectives

As a manager or supervisor you may need to **prioritise** the identified team and individual needs because of financial and time constraints.

To do

■ Make a list of each one then compare it with the individual job descriptions and the team development needs.

Team and organisational **values** may be different from the **training needs**, for example an organisational value may be that the salon always closes on Sunday, but the training need may be that a full day's staff training can only be delivered on a Sunday.

To do

■ List three different organisational values against three different training needs.

Once all the team and individual needs have been identified you may need to gain agreement from

- **Team members**
- **Other managers** or colleagues working at the same level
- **Line managers** (above your level)
- **Specialists** (such as manufacturer's trainers)

You will need to use your prioritised list of training and list the strengths and weaknesses of each. For example:

Individual training needs

Strengths:
- Implementing model nights for junior staff
- Implementing long-hair training sessions for all staff
- Managing a full client column

Appraisal Questionnaire*

Name of Appraisee   *Rachel Davies*   Job Title   *Senior Stylist*

Name of Appraiser   *Stephanie Henderson*   Line Manager   *Noel Otley*

Date appointed to present post   *September 1997*

Appraisal Cycle From   *November 1999*   to   *November 2000*

Current work & responsibilities

Staff Trainer
Attends to clients
Long hair specialist

Which areas of work are you least satisfied with?

Time Management
Negative feedback from some juniors when criticised during training

What objectives or goals have been achieved in the last appraisal cycle?

Fully booked client column 3 weeks in advance
Planned and reviewed model nights for juniors
Presented 3 long hair training sessions for staff

What objectives or goals are still to be achieved?

To review and prepare a report on the client questionnaire
To include hair extensions as a salon service
To improve my time management
To improve feedback during training the junior staff

What action needs to be done to achieve them?

To collate all questionnaires and extract the strengths and weaknesses
To attend training in hair extensions for both synthetic and real hair
To attend a time management course
To attain D32 D33 TDLB training certificate

What other achievements have been made?

Attended a first aid course and achieved Life Savers Certificate – St Johns Ambulance Brigade
Attended three manufacturers courses to update colour, perm and cutting skills

* A blank photocopiable version of this form appears on pages 250 and 251.

Objectives/Goals to be achieved within this appraisal cycle

Objectives/Goals	Action	Criteria for Success	Time Scale
To prepare a report from the client questionnaire	To collate all questionnaires and extract the strengths and weaknesses	Complete report based on questionnaires	End of Jan 2000
To offer hair extensions as a salon service	To attend a hair extension course and become competent	Hair extension Diploma	End of March 2000
To improve my time management	To attend a time management training course	Decrease in client waiting time reviewed through client questionnaires	End of June 2000
To attain TDLB D32/D33 Training Certificate	To register with a local college and City & Guilds, attend training courses and complete the work	D32/D33 Certificates	End of October 2000

Personal Development Plan

What are your career objectives?

To become a salon manager within the next three years
To increase my client takings by 20%

What additional training/knowledge/skills are needed by the appraisee?

Guidance with preparing client questionnaire report
To practice in the use of hair extensions on a tuition head
To be able to transfer time management knowledge to a client column
To understand the amount of work required to obtain D32/D33 Certificate

What actions need to be taken to meet these training needs?

To discuss client questionnaire with line manager
To research the cost of hair extensions for practice
To prepare a list of questions regarding client columns to take to the time management course
To discuss the course requirements of obtaining D32/D33 with my local college tutor

Comment by Appraiser	Comment by Appraiser's Line Manager
Excellent achievements, well done	Well done, we will try to help fund most of your new training needs
Signature S. Henderson Date 10/11/99	Signature N Otley Date 18/11/99

Comment by Appraisee	Signature and date of Appraiser when returned
Thanks for being so helpful, I can't wait to start	25/11/99 S Henderson
	Signature and date of Appraisee when returned
Signature R Davies Date 12/11/99	26/11/99 R Davies

Weaknesses:
- Unable to offer hair extension services to clients
- Coping with negative feedback from some junior staff in training
- Running late with appointment system

Team training needs

Strengths:
- Well motivated and enthusiastic team members
- All staff trained to a minimum of NVQ L2 standards
- Ongoing training by a specific manufacturer in current products

Weaknesses:
- No staff able to offer hair extension services
- Client waiting time increased due to poor time management
- Assessment feedback techniques causing ill feeling amongst some trainees

Integrating appraisals into development planning needs

A good development plan needs to utilise appraisals, and the following are examples of training that could take place:

- Hair extension training for one member of staff to cascade to others (to a specialist such as a manufacturer's trainer and to team members)
- Time management training for key members of staff (to a line manager)
- TDLB D32 D33 training for the staff trainer (to colleagues working at the same level)

Organisational constraints

The salon's developmental planning needs may be at odds with the organisational constraints – e.g.:

- **Time** – salons are busiest at holiday times and staff training may be better taken at quiet periods
- **Finance** – the salon's training budget could be enhanced by sponsorship from a manufacturer
- **Line management** – senior staff may be intimidated by junior staff offering specialist training, therefore a senior member may need the initial training to cascade to others

Implementing development plans

To ensure equal access by enabling every member of your team to be involved, development plans must take account of

- **Team members' work activities** – e.g. a training evening after a busy day when staff are tired is not as beneficial as using a period when the salon is quiet.
- **Team members' learning abilities** – e.g. it is not beneficial to give advanced training to junior staff who have not completed their initial training.
- **Team members' personal circumstances** – e.g. staff who have a long distance to travel to work may not be able to attend an early morning training session.

> **Remember**
>
> All development plans must be agreed with everyone involved to create harmony and a positive communication system.

To do

■ List three other reasons why you should consider the above points.

The manager's contributions

There are three ways in which you could contribute personally towards planning developments.

- By taking part in the development activity yourself through issuing briefing documents e.g.

Memo

To   All Staff
From   Stephanie Henderson - contact extension 223 re any
        queries
Date   27/11/99
Re   **Staff training Session on long hair**
        Wednesday evening 06/01/00 6.30pm – 8.30pm
All staff are required to bring one model at 6.30pm with
hair below shoulder length which has been washed the day
previously.
The salon will supply pins, grips and ornamentation. We will
continue to practice for our bridal theme.
Looking forward to seeing you there.
Signed
                S Henderson
            Stephanie Henderson

- By providing opportunities for learning at work, e.g.

Notice to all Staff

Client Questionnaire

Please ensure that each of your clients is given the opportunity to complete the enclosed sample of the client questionnaire form during the forthcoming week. Please place the completed forms in the box by reception.

We shall analyse the results to decide if we need to provide any further staff training in customer service.

Please call me on extension 223 if you have any problems or queries.

From Stephanie Henderson

Manager

- By modifying development activities to take account of the feedback you have received, e.g.

Memo

To   All Staff
From   Stephanie Henderson - contact extension 223 re any
        queries
Date   28/11/99
Re   **Staff training on long hair**
The salon's appointment book is becoming too busy to hold
this session on the date arranged yesterday – and this has
been confirmed by memos from several staff members. I have
therefore rescheduled the training day for 8th January.
Please make a note of this in your diaries.

Signed   *S Henderson*
            Stephanie Henderson

Choosing the development activity

Different development activities, such as offering hair extensions as a salon service, improving time management, obtaining TDLB qualifications, need different considerations before any decisions to go ahead can be made.

- **The team members:**
  - Is the activity suitable for their clientele?
  - Would they need considerable practice?
- **The type of development activity:**
  - Is it cost effective?
  - Is it time effective?
- **The manager's own abilities:**
  - Is training needed beforehand in organisational or motivational skills?
- **The situation:**
  - Is there enough space in the salon for the training?
  - Will there be enough suitable models for the training?

Once all these factors have been considered:

- Provision of information – e.g. from the appraisals and client question-naires
- Instructions – e.g. from a Health and Safety Policy document
- Skills and training – e.g. hair extensions
- Provision of learning opportunities at work – e.g. training in long hair

through discussions with all staff personnel, then time must be allowed for **feedback** (evident in the memos or notices to staff) **before implementation**.

Presenting ideas for planning developments

The ideas that have been gathered from **individual appraisals**, **results of client surveys**, **informal and formal staff meetings** and **published literature** about available **training** courses must be collated and prioritised for formal presentations.

Initially **agreement** should be gained from the **authorised people** – i.e. the training personnel involved, then the higher level line manager. Colleagues at the same level should then be informed and, finally, to the rest of the team.

When agreement has been gained from all those involved then the development plan can be implemented.

The assessment of development objectives

Reviews are important in the development planning process because they will enable the manager to focus on whether knowledge and skills and performance at work have **improved** by looking at the **success criteria** of the stated **goals and objectives**.

Improvement may be measured by

- **Testing knowledge or skills** through identifying agreed criteria – e.g. attaining D32/D33 TDLB assessors awards
- **Observation of performance at work** – e.g. analysing the client's questionnaires regarding waiting times.
- **Appraisal discussions** – by completing an appraisal review document

Staff can contribute to their own progress by taking part in an appraisal review, making any comments and signing to say that the review is valid.

Salon personnel must be confident that all assessments are **confidential** and that documents are available only to **authorised people**. This would help to create harmony in the team.

All assessment results should be discussed with the individuals or teams being assessed, then the higher level line manager, then (if appropriate) colleagues working at the same level as the manager, and finally with any specialists involved.

Remedial actions

Hopefully, by using the effective communication techniques described in this chapter, you will have given constructive feedback and have a happy, motivated work team. However, problems can happen. For instance:

1. You have allocated someone a training job and they have not carried it out at all

There are two possible solutions to this:

- You must reallocate the training work to someone of equal competence.
- You need to counsel the person and explain how important it was that the job was done, and then refer the matter to your immediate manager. **This must be done privately – never in front of other staff**.

2. You have allocated someone a training job and they have not carried it out in the way you specified

The usual reason for this is that you did not explain the job clearly enough. The answer is therefore to provide more support by explaining it again, giving the person some instructions to read, or by asking someone else to demonstrate the skill to them again.

Appraisal Review*

Name of Appraisee   *Rachel Davies*

Job Title   *Senior Stylist*

Date of Review   *June 2000*

Review of Objectives Set

Objectives which have been achieved should be listed. Where objectives have been changed new ones should be agreed. All objectives should be achievable and measurable.

Objectives/Goals	Action	Criteria for Success	Time Scale
To prepare a report from the client questionnaire	*To collate all questionnaires and extract the strengths and weaknesses*	*Complete report based on questionnaires*	*End of Jan 2000*
To offer hair extensions as a salon service	*To attend a hair extension course and become competent*	*Hair extension Diploma*	*End of March 2000*
To improve my time management	*To attend a time management training course*	*Decrease in client waiting time reviewed through client questionnaires*	*End of June 2000*
To attain TDLB D32/D33 Training Certificate	*To register with a local college and City & Guilds, attend on training courses and complete the work*	*D32/D33 Certificates*	*End of October 2000*

Review of Training Development Needs

Training development carried out by appraisee since last review

Direction regarding preparing client questionnaire summary results from line manager
Attended hair extension course in February 2000
Enrolled and attended local college to attain D32/D33 certification

Training and development requirements which have been changed since last review

Time management issue now being resolved through closer supervision of client appointment schedules

Action which will be taken to meet changed requirements

Discussion forum with all staff personnel to analyse client timings for the appointment schedules

* A blank photocopiable version of this form appears on pages 252 and 253.

Criteria used to assess whether training and development which takes place is a success

Client surveys indicated that some staff need to obtain customer service NVQ
Hair extension services utilised by clients
3 summative assessments obtained towards D32/D33 certification

Comments by Appraiser

You have worked very hard in all areas and are achieving your planned goals.

Signature   *S Henderson*   Date   *10/11/99*

Comments by Appraisee

I am pleased with my attainments to date and hope to complete my D32 D33 by September 2000

Signature   *R Davies*   Date   *12/6/00*

Comments by Appraiser's Line Manager

Very good achievements, you have also helped the team development by highlighting both reception and customer care development needs. Well done.

Signature   *N Otley*   Date   *26/6/00*

Test your knowledge

1 Why is it important to encourage salon personnel to develop **effective salon improvements**?
2 How can the **manager** or **supervisor contribute** towards these improvements?
3 Why should you provide **salon personnel** with opportunities to **contribute** to identifying their **own development needs**?
4 Describe the **differences** between **development needs** which may meet **team objectives** and those which meet **individual aspirations**.
5 How can the **manager** or **supervisor prioritise** between **team** development needs and **individual** aspirational development needs?
6 Describe the **implications** of comparing **team** development **values** with team development **training needs**.
7 How could you present **development needs** in a **positive way** to the following:
- **Team members**
- **Colleagues** working at the same level
- **Line managers**
- **Specialists**?
8 What are the principles of **good practice** in planning the development of teams and individuals?

continued

Test your knowledge *continued*

9   Describe how an **appraisal system** can be integrated into the salon's developmental planning needs.

10   List two **organisational constraints** that may influence the salon's **developmental planning needs** and describe how they could be incorporated into the **planning process**.

11   Why and how do development plans have to be **agreed** with everyone involved?

12   Why should **developmental plans** take **account** of
   ■ Team members' **work activities**
   ■ Team members' **learning abilities**
   ■ Team members' **personal circumstances**
and how could you take these into account?

13   List **three different contributions** the manager can make to the various activities for team members.

14   How could the manager decide on what **contributions** to make towards developmental activities relating to
   ■ The **team members**
   ■ The type of **developmental activity**
   ■ The **manager's own abilities**
   ■ The **situation**?

15   How could the manager ensure that **their own contribution** is meeting the **agreed objectives and plans**?

16   How and why should the manager monitor and review development activities and note the **feedback** of those taking part?

17   What are the **correct procedures** for **presenting ideas** and contributions to planning developments?

18   Why is it important to **assess team members'** development?

19   Why should the **range of purposes of an assessment** be agreed with all salon personal and specialists?

20   State the reasons why **team members** should contribute towards the assessment of **their own progress**, giving examples of how this could be done.

21   Describe the principles of **objective and fair assessment**.

22   Detail how you could implement the following assessment methods objectively and fairly:
   ■ Testing of **knowledge and skills**
   ■ **Observation of performance at work**
   ■ **Appraisal discussions**.

23   Why is **confidentiality** important during assessment procedures?

24   Describe the **procedures** for reporting **assessment results**.

Appendix:

Salon forms and records

You may photocopy these forms for personal use.

Contents

Example Time and Motion Study

Week beginning:

	SERVICES				
	Cut and blow dry	Blow dry/set	Perm	Colour	Relaxer
Time allocated*:					
Day/date					
Totals for week:					
Time spent (hours)					

*average time for basic perm/realxing/colouring techniques – not including processing or drying time

Number of hours worked:

Health and Safety Policy Review Dates

	Planned date	Actual review
1		
2		
3		
4		
5		
6		
7		
8		
9		
10		
11		
12		
13		
14		
15		
16		
17		
18		
19		
20		

Health and Safety Policy: Important Contacts

Key contact	Contact name	Tel/fax	Address
Environmental Health Officer			
Hospital			
Doctor			
Fire Safety Officer			
Employment Medical Advisory Service			
Local Police Station			

Salon Rules

Salon safety and hygiene

Fixtures, fittings, chairs, trolleys and mirrors to be regularly cleaned.

Non-electrical equipment to be kept clean and sterilised at all times.

Electrical equipment to be visually checked for safety, then switched off, unplugged and stored between use.

Floors to be swept clean, free from hair, and spillages immediately mopped up.

Used gowns and towels to be placed in the laundry basket.

Rubbish to be removed immediately and placed in a covered container. Store in sealed rubbish bags while awaiting disposal.

Food and drink must be consumed only in the staff rest room.

Rest room to be kept clean and tidy. Wash up cups, plates and saucers immediately after use.

Staff who smoke must use the smoking area in the rest room.

Stock room to be kept clean and tidy. Stock to be correctly stored and lids and tops replaced immediately after use.

Reception area to be kept clean and tidy.

Fire precautions

Smoking is not allowed in any area of the salon, only outside the back entrance.

Keep all fire exits and egress to them clear at all times.

Do not obstruct fire extinguishers.

Unlock fire exits during working hours.

Security

Keep till drawer locked when not in use.

Keep all stock doors and cupboards locked when not in use.

Do not bring any valuables to the salon. Keep your purse/money on your person at all times.

Lock all fire exits, close all windows and lock all doors at night.

FIRE DRILL

IN THE EVENT OF A FIRE:

1. TELEPHONE 999 FOR THE FIRE BRIGADE

2. CLOSE ALL DOORS AND WINDOWS

3. LEAVE THE BUILDING BY THE NEAREST EXIT

4. ASSEMBLE OUTSIDE THE SALON

DO NOT:

1. STOP TO COLLECT ANY PERSONAL BELONGINGS

2. RE-ENTER THE BUILDING UNTIL THE ALL-CLEAR HAS BEEN GIVEN

THE NEAREST EXITS ARE:

THE SALON FRONT DOOR

THE SALON BACK DOOR

IF YOU FIND AN
UNATTENDED PARCEL, A SUSPICIOUS OBJECT,
OR IF YOU SUSPECT THAT THERE IS LIKELY TO
BE AN **EXPLOSIVE DEVICE, GAS LEAK**, ETC. IN
OR NEAR THE SALON

- **DO NOT TOUCH OR MOVE THE PARCEL/OBJECT**

- **EVACUATE THE SALON**

- **CALL THE POLICE**

- **WARN MEMBERS OF THE PUBLIC**

- **WARN THE OCCUPANTS OF ADJACENT PREMISES**

DO NOT RE-ENTER THE AREA UNTIL
INSTRUCTED TO DO SO BY THE POLICE

ALWAYS REMEMBER

IF IN DOUBT – SHOUT!

Health and Safety Risk Evaluation

Potential hazard	Degree of risk High/Med/Low (please circle)	Persons at risk	Action needed to minimise risk	By when	By whom
1	L M H				
2	L M H				
3	L M H				
4	L M H				
5	L M H				
6	L M H				

Health and Safety Training Record

Staff name	Staff signature	Health and Safety policy and Salon Rules	Fire precautions	First aid and accidents	COSSH	Personal protective equipment	Electrical equipment	Trainer's signature	Review dates					

Areas inducted

Health and Safety Induction Questionnaire

Name _____   *Date* _____

1.   Who is the main person in charge of Health and Safety in the salon?

_____

2.   Who is responsible for day-to-day Health and Safety?

_____

3.   Who does the Health and Safety training?

_____

4.   Who is in charge of:

		Person responsible	*Salon location*
a)	Salon Rules	_____	_____
b)	First Aid Box	_____	_____
c)	Accident Book	_____	_____
d)	COSHH assessments	_____	_____
e)	Personal Protective Equipment	_____	_____
f)	Fire drills	_____	_____
g)	Notices	_____	_____
h)	Exit signs	_____	_____

Health and Safety Induction Questionnaire (Contd.)

5.   Describe the different fire extinguishers:

Colour	Type	Use
_____	_____	_____
_____	_____	_____
_____	_____	_____
_____	_____	_____
_____	_____	_____
_____	_____	_____

Schedule of Electrical Items

Item	Serial no.	Purchase date	Disposal date
1			
2			
3			
4			
5			
6			
7			
8			
9			
10			
11			
12			

Testing Programme for Salon Appliances

ELECTRICAL SUPPLIER			TESTING DATES						
Name and address	Tel. No.		Target	Actual	Target	Actual	Target	Actual	

COSSH Risk Assessment

Hazard	What is the risk?	Degree of risk			Who is at risk?	Action to be taken	Date
		High	Med	Low			

Fire Equipment Test Record

| FIRE EQUIPMENT SUPPLIER | | TESTING DATES | | | | | |
Name and address	Tel. No.	Target	Actual	Target	Actual	Target	Actual

Accident Book

When did the accident happen? (Give date and time)	Where did the accident happen?	How did the accident happen? (Give as much detail as possible)	Name of person(s) involved and nature of injuries	Who investigated and reported the accident? (Give full name and position)	Was the accident reportable under RIDDOR?

Asthma/Dermatitis Records

Name	Reported date of symptoms	Description of symptoms	Date and results of medical advice	Precautions required

Routine Health and Safety Checks

Inspection items/area	Staff member responsible	Inspection dates/initials							
Safety inspections									
Enforcing salon rules									
Inspecting electrical equipment									
First Aid kit									
Accident Book									
Fire exits/extinguishers/fire drills/assembly points									
Day-to-day Health and Safety									
COSHH Assessments									

Hair and Beauty Show Evaluation

Please spare two minutes to complete this questionnaire to let us know how you felt about the show.

Please tick the *Yes* or *No* boxes:

		Yes	No
1.	Did you enjoy the show?	☐	☐
2.	Could you see everything clearly?	☐	☐
3.	Could you hear everything that was said?	☐	☐
4.	Did you find it easy to purchase the tickets?	☐	☐
5.	Was the Level 2 (full-time students') work up to the standard you expected?	☐	☐
6.	Was the Level 3 (mature students') work up to the standard you expected?	☐	☐
7.	Did you find the college map helpful?	☐	☐
8.	Was the price of the ticket good value for money?	☐	☐
9.	Were the refreshments sufficient?	☐	☐
10.	If we put on another show next year, will you come again?	☐	☐

Please feel free to add any other comments below:

_____

Name _____

Signature _____   Date _____

Candidate Appraisal Form

Name _____

Date _____

	Supervisor's Grading		*Supervisor's Grading*
Attendance	☐	Cutting	☐
Punctuality	☐	Setting	☐
Attitude to work	☐	Blow-drying	☐
Attitude to group	☐	Perming	☐
Attitude to clients	☐	Colouring	☐
Personal presentation	☐		
Written assignment marks	☐		

Candidate response

_____

_____

Signature _____

Supervisor's comments

_____

_____

Signature _____

Grading: **A** – Excellent **B** – Very Good **C** – Good **D** – Average **E** – Poor

Client Questionnaire

In our salon you, the client, are the most important person. We would therefore like to improve our service to you and would appreciate a few moments of your time to complete this simple questionnaire.

Date   _____

Service required   _____

Area where you live   _____

Your age group   15–25 / 35–45 / 45–60 / 60+

     (please circle)

What time of day?   9 am–12 pm / 12 pm–2 pm / 2 pm–6 pm / 6 pm–9 pm

Was your service   Excellent/Good/Average/Poor?

Were you given a free consultation?   Yes/No

Was the salon up to your standard of cleanliness?   Yes/No

What was the attitude of the staff that attended to you?

     Excellent/Good/Average/Poor

Did you have to wait for any part of your service?   Yes/No

(if applicable) Was the waiting time acceptable to you?   Yes/No

Are you happy with the quality of service offered at our salon?   Yes/No

Do you consider our salon gives good value for money?   Yes/No

Are you dissatisfied with any part of the services offered?   Yes/No

If yes, briefly describe what was wrong

_____

Client Questionnaire (Contd.)

Would you like any additional hairdressing or beauty services offered in the salon?   Yes/No

If yes, please describe.

_____

If you are a new client, will you return to us?   Yes/No

If no, why not?

_____

If you are a regular client, what is it that keeps you coming to us?

_____

Is there any particular member of staff you find outstanding?   Yes/No

If yes, who is it?

_____

Please place the questionnaire in the box by reception as you leave.

Many thanks

Pre-Appraisal Questionnaire

Name of Appraisee
Job Title

Current work & responsibilities

Objectives achieved and outstanding objectives

Which areas of work are you least satisfied with?

What topics or issues would you like to discuss?

Development Needs

What skills do you feel need to be developed further?

What particular training do you require?

Name   Signature   Date

Appraisal Questionnaire

Name of Appraisee   Job Title

Name of Appraiser   Line Manager

Date appointed to present post

Appraisal Cycle From   to

Current work & responsibilities

Which areas of work are you least satisfied with?

What objectives or goals have been achieved in the last appraisal cycle?

What objectives or goals are still to be achieved?

What action needs to be done to achieve them?

What other achievements have been made?

Objectives/Goals to be achieved within this appraisal cycle

Objectives/Goals	Action	Criteria for Success	Time Scale

Personal Development Plan

What are your career objectives?

What additional training/knowledge/skills are needed by the appraisee?

What actions need to be taken to meet these training needs?

Comment by Appraiser	Comment by Appraiser's Line Manager
Signature Date	Signature Date

Comment by Appraisee	Signature and date of Appraiser when returned
	Signature and date of Appraisee when returned
Signature Date	

Appraisal Review

Name of Appraisee

Job Title

Date of Review

Review of Objectives Set

Objectives which have been achieved should be listed. Where objectives have been changed new ones should be agreed. All objectives should be achievable and measurable.

Objectives/Goals	Action	Criteria for Success	Time Scale

Review of Training Development Needs

Training development carried out by appraisee since last review

Training and development requirements which have been changed since last review

Action which will be taken to meet changed requirements

Criteria used to assess whether training and development which takes place is a success

Comments by Appraiser

Signature   Date

Comments by Appraisee

Signature   Date

Comments by Appraiser's Line Manager

Signature   Date

APL Evidence Summary Sheet

Candidate's name: Award title: Assessor's name:

Unit or element claimed	Listing of experience	References and CV	Product evidence	Certificates and awards

Interview notes	Other evidence	Top-up training needed	Sufficient valid evidence

Candidate's signature   Date assessment plan agreed

Assessor's signature   Date of assessment

Candidate Practical Action Plan

Name   _____

Start date   _____

Date   _____   Candidate signature

Target elements   _____

Target date   _____   _____

Comments   _____

     Assessor signature

_____

_____   _____

Date   _____   Candidate signature

Target elements   _____

Target date   _____   _____

Comments

_____   Assessor signature

_____   _____

_____

_____

Line Management Chart

Name	Position	Experience and qualification	Limits of authority

Example Assessment Plan

Candidate name _____

Assessor _____

Unit no. and title _____

Element no. and title _____

Approximate timing of assessment _____

Evidence to be presented

Natural performance in the workplace ☐   Records of prior achievement ☐

Responses to oral questions ☐   Reports from colleagues ☐

Written projects and assignments ☐   Reports from supervisors in workplaces ☐

Review of written records e.g. client record cards ☐   Simulated work activities ☐

Completed assessment question papers ☐   Other evidence of competency ☐

Details

People involved in my assessment

Assessor ☐
Clients ☐
Supervisor ☐
Others ☐

Special assessment requirements and issues I need to agree with the people concerned

_____

_____

Schedule for assessment and review

Date: Date: Date:
Purpose: Purpose: Purpose:

_____   _____   _____

Candidate signature   Date plan agreed   Assessor signature

_____   _____   _____

Index